Graft-versus-Host Disease - Natural History and Prevention Levels

Edited by Nicolás Padilla-Raygoza and Eunice Sandoval Ramírez

Published in London, United Kingdom

IntechOpen

intechopen.com

Built by scientists, for scientists

Meet the editors

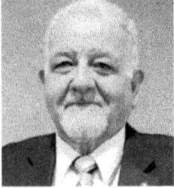

Dr. Nicolás Padilla-Raygoza was Professor Titular B at the University of Guanajuato, México, and Coordinator of Research at the University of Celaya, México. He is currently the coordinator of research projects at the Institute of Public Health in the state of Guanajuato. He obtained an MD from Universidad Autónoma de Guadalajara and University Autonomous of México in 1984, specialization in pediatrics from the Mexican Council of Certification in 1986, a postgraduate degree in Epidemiology from the University of London in 2001, a master's degree and doctorate in Science from Atlantic International University in 2006, and a master's degree in Social Gerontology from the International Iberoamerican University in 2017. He has 190 journal articles and 59 book chapters to his credit. He has also edited five books on health. He was recognized as a state researcher in health by the Institute of Public Health of Guanajuato State in 2015 and as a researcher with social impact by Urbanizadora del Bajío, S. A. in 2016. He is a member of the National Researchers System in México.

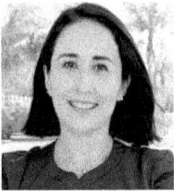

Dra. Eunice Sandoval-Ramírez, originally from Guerrero, is a surgeon at the National Autonomous University of Mexico, specializing in Pediatric Allergy and Immunology. She graduated from the National Institute of Pediatrics and the "Federico Gómez" Children's Hospital of Mexico. She currently practices at the Angeles Leon Hospital and is an Immunology professor at La Salle University in Bajio.

Contents

Preface

With the increasing use of hematopoietic stem cell transplants as a treatment for malignancies and other pathologies, the frequency of graft-versus-host disease (GVHD) has increased. GVHD can be observed after allogeneic hematopoietic stem cell transplantation and can present in acute and chronic forms; the acute form has an incidence of 30% to 50% in (allogeneic) hematopoietic stem cell transplants, and in transplants from haploidentical-matched unrelated donors, being reported before 100 days after transplantation, and the chronic form appears after 100 days after transplantation.

Chronic GVHD is the leading cause of death, not due to relapse of the original disease, and may evolve from acute to chronic, quiescent (acute GVHD that resolves but later develops into chronic form) or may occur de novo.

It was decided to utilize the natural history of the disease and its prevention levels to review GVHD, as this is a unique approach to evaluating any type of pathology. This book covers the pre-pathogenic period, also known as the ecological triad, which includes the agent, host, and environment prior to the development of the disease. Clinical manifestations of the different types of GVHD are also included. Regarding prevention levels, sanitary education and health promotion, specific protection, and various treatments for the disease are reviewed. The editors and authors of the chapters hope that you find the chapters useful for your education and health practice.

The editors recognize the hard work of the authors and are grateful for the tremendous support of Mirna Papuga, Publishing Process Manager, from IntechOpen.

Dr. Nicolás Padilla-Raygoza
Department of Research and Technological Development,
Directorate of Teaching and Research,
Institute of Public Health from Guanajuato State,
Guanajuato, Mexico

Dra. Eunice Sandoval-Ramírez
Professor,
La Salle University in Bajio,
Guanajuato, Mexico

Chapter 1

Pre-Pathogenic Period: Ecological Triad of Graft-Versus-Host Disease

Nicolás Padilla-Raygoza, Eunice Sandoval Ramírez,
Gilberto Flores-Vargas, María de Jesús Gallardo-Luna
and Efraín Navarro-Olivos

Abstract

There is an increase in diseases that are treated with hematopoietic stem cell, bone marrow, or/and organ transplants. The frequency of graft-versus-host disease and its risk factors that promote the presence of the disease are reviewed. The agent is the presence of T cells in the transplanted cells or organs, and the host does not mount an effective immune response against them or the medical treatment to prevent the immune response was not effective. The host who suffers from graft-versus-host disease is any person who receives cell or organ transplants for any underlying disease that can be treated with transplant. Regarding the environment, no factors have been described that may influence the presence of graft-versus-host disease. It is important to balance the elements of the ecological triad (agent-host-environment), so that graft-versus-host disease does not occur. The important thing is that the person with a disorder that requires hematopoietic stem cells, marrow or organ transplant, receive a prophylactic scheme to avoid the immune response against the transplant.

Keywords: agent, host, environment, transplant, hematopoietic stem cell

1. Introduction

The disease process is dynamic, and reviewing it in the form of natural history and levels of disease prevention allows for a didactic way of learning about the evaluation of a pathology and how to prevent it at different stages. The ecological triad in pre-pathogenic period only includes agent, host, and environment, before that the disease is in the person, but has relationship with pathogenic period and prevention levels (**Table 1**).

Organ, bone marrow, and hematopoietic cell transplants are increasingly used worldwide as a treatment for many malignant and non-malignant diseases, and these treatments are often the only way to cure these diseases.

Hematopoietic stem cell transplantation (HSCT) is a potentially curative treatment for malignancies such as leukemia, lymphoma, myeloma, and myelodysplasia, but also for non-malignant diseases such as hemoglobinopathies, aplastic anemia, and immunodeficiency syndromes (inborn errors of immunity [1, 2]); due to the increase

IntechOpen

Pre-pathogenic period-ecological triad		Pathogenic period		
Agent: presence of T cells in blood, marrow, or organ transplanted. Host: patients that require bloods stem cell, marrow, or organ transplants and generate an immune response to T cells present in the transplant from donor.		Complications → Sequelae → Recovery → Death Clinical stage Clinical horizon		
Environment: without evidence of relationship with graft-versus-host disease, but there is an association with subjacent diseases		Subclinical stage (physiopathology)		
Primary prevention		Secondary prevention		Tertiary prevention
First level Sanitary education and health promotion	Second level Specific protection	Third level (early diagnosis and timely treatment)	Fourth level Limitation of damage (treatment of complications)	Fifth level Rehabilitation

CH Clinical horizon.
Source: Own design.

Table 1.
Natural history of disease and prevention levels.

in the prevalence of these diseases and timely diagnosis, offering the possibility of access to definitive treatment, the number of hematopoietic cell transplants has also increased [3].

Prior to HSCT, patients undergo chemotherapy to eradicate affected hematologic cells, provide an immunosuppressive environment for the transplanted cells, and prevent rejection of the donor hematopoietic cells to be transplanted [2].

For graft-versus-host disease (GVHD), a frequency of 40–80% is reported after transplantation of marrow and blood replete with T cells [4, 5].

GVHD can be observed after allogeneic hematopoietic stem cell transplantation and can present in acute and chronic forms; the acute form has an incidence of 30–50% in allogeneic hematopoietic stem cell transplants (a-HSCT) [6] and in transplants from matched haploidentical unrelated donors [6, 7], and being reported before 100 days after transplantation and the chronic form appears after 100 days after transplantation [8, 9].

Despite significant advances in donor selection, conditioning regimens, and prophylaxis, chronic GVHD remains the major cause of late morbidity and mortality [10].

National Institutes of Health criteria have been used to classify GVHD into four subclasses [11]:

1. Classic acute graft-versus- host disease (aGVHD): Presentation within 100 days of transplantation or donor lymphocyte infusion,

2. Late-onset persistent and/or recurrent aGVHD: Features of classic aGVHD without diagnostic manifestations of chronic graft-versus-host disease (cGVHD) occurring beyond 100 days after transplantation,

3. Classic cGVHD: Diagnostic and distinctive features of cGVHD are present and presenting after 100 days

4. Overlap syndrome: Features of both cGVHD and aGVHD may be observed.

The cGVHD is the leading cause of death not due to relapse of the original disease [12] and may be the evolution from acute to chronic, quiescent (aGVHD that resolves but later the chronic form appears) or may occur de *novo* [13].

The two leading causes of death after allogenic HSCT are relapse of the underlying disease and GVHD [14].

2. Ecological triad

For the presentation of GVHD, three conditions are necessary, according to Billingham [15]:

1. The donor/graft must contain immunologically competent cells.

2. The recipient/host must express tissue antigens that are not present in the donated cells; and

3. The recipient must be unable to establish an immunologically effective response to eliminate the transplanted cells.

Host tissue antigens are presented to donor T cells, which activate them and initiate an immune response against the host with the secretion of inflammatory cytokines such as tumor necrosis factor-alpha (TNF-alpha) and interleukins 1 (IL-1) and 6 (IL-6) [16].

2.1 Agent

GVHD is caused by the presence of T cells in transplanted organs, marrow, or blood, and the recipient is unable to mount an immunologically effective response to eliminate those donor T cells [17, 18], or prophylaxis to prevent the immune response with cyclosporine, methotrexate, or steroids was not effective [19].

The donor T cell recognition response that induces GVHD is mostly directed against the host major histocompatibility complex (HMHC) or mismatches between minor histocompatibility antigens (MHA) [20]. Recognition of mismatches in the polymorphic MHC class I chain-related gene A or MICA is a factor for the development of GVHD [21].

This immune response with release of proinflammatory cytokines induces pathophysiological changes that will lead to the clinical form of GVHD, in the form of immunocompetent effector T lymphocytes responding to polymorphic and non-polymorphic antigens of the donor/recipient with activation, inflammation, and cytolytic activity [22].

2.2 Host

For GVHD to occur, the person must have undergone a bone marrow or hemato-poietic cell transplant. Theoretically, it could also occur in organ transplants.

The host at risk for GVHD is patients who have malignancies or any disease requiring transplants and whose prophylactic regimen to prevent this immune response has been ineffective.

Risk factors for developing GVHD are [23]:

- Peripheral hematopoietic cells with mobilized growth factor,

- Unrelated or mismatched donor grafts,

- Sex disparity between donor and recipient, i.e., female to male transplant or vice versa,

- Recipient with advanced age,

- Intensity of the conditioning regimen,

- Multiparous female donor [19].

For this to occur, Antin and Ferrara [24] described a three-step process for the development of GVHD:

    i. Host tissue damage with production of inflammatory cytokines,

    ii. Stimulation and production of effector T cells (Teff); and

    iii. Recruitment and activation of mononuclear effectors and amplification of the cytokine storm.

Immune reconstitution after HSCT may result in:

    i. Natural immune restoration of protective immunity with host tolerance,

    ii. Functional tolerance with anti-graft pathology effects, or

    iii. Dysregulation and alloreactivity causing aGVHD or later cGVHD [25].

Another important aspect is glucose metabolism which plays an important role in inflammation [26], and glycolysis is essential for T cell activation, supporting their growth and proliferation [27]. Increased glycolytic activity has been reported in T cells when activated by allo-antigens [28]. Therefore, patients with impaired glucose metabolism undergoing HSCT will be at risk of developing GVHD.

Activated AMP-protein kinase has been reported to be a driver of oxidative metabolism, restricting anabolism and promoting catabolic pathways including oxidative phosphorylation and autophagy [29]. Increased AMPK phosphorylation has been found in alloreactive T cells, and genetic deletion of AMPK in donor T cells showed a protective effect against GVHD [30].

2.3 Environment

There is no evidence of environmental factors that are considered for the presentation of GVHD, although there is evidence for the development of pathologies that led to the development of the original disease, which led to hematopoietic cell transplantation.

In Mexico, in a study of patients who underwent allogeneic hematopoietic cell transplantation, they did not find that geographic factors were a risk factor for GVHD [31].

Gómez-De León et al. [31] report that access to private insurance coverage for allogenic HSCT showed an association with improved survival and reduced mortality not due to relapse.

3. Conclusion

The main way to prevent GVHD is to prevent people from developing the diseases for which HSCT is needed, so that the ecological triad remains balanced.

For those who have already developed these diseases, they should avoid the agent and host factors that lead to GVHD.

The balance between the agent, the host, and the environment maintains the health of the individual, and the appearance of GVHD will be delayed.

If the patient receives HBST, marrow or organ transplant, they should be managed with a chemoprophylaxis regimen to avoid the immune response to transplant.

Conflict of interest

The authors declare no conflict of interest.

Author details

Nicolás Padilla-Raygoza[1]*, Eunice Sandoval Ramírez[2], Gilberto Flores-Vargas[1], María de Jesús Gallardo-Luna[1] and Efraín Navarro-Olivos[3]

1 Department of Research and Technological Development, Teaching and Research, Institute of Public Health from Guanajuato State, Guanajuato, Mexico

2 Immunology, School of Medicine, University Lasalle, León, Mexico

3 Teaching and Research, Institute of Public Health from Guanajuato State, Guanajuato, Mexico

*Address all correspondence to: npadillar@guanajuato.gob.mx

IntechOpen

References

[1] Notarangelo LD, Bacchetta R, Casanova JL, Su HC. Human inborn errors of immunity: An expanding universe. Science Immunology. 2020;**5**(49):eabb1662. DOI: 10.1126/sciimmunol.abb1662

[2] Gratwhol A, Baldomero H, Aljurf M. Hematopoietic stem cell transplantation: A global perspective. Journal of the American Medical Association. 2010;**303**:1617-1624. DOI: 10.1001/jama.2010.491

[3] Hamilton BK. Updates in chronic graft-versus-host disease. Hematology. American Society of Hematology. Education Program. 2021;**2021**(1):648-654. DOI: 10.1182/hematology.2021000301

[4] MacMillan ML, Weisdorf DJ, Wagner JE, DeFor TE, Burns LJ, Ramsay NKC, et al. Response of 443 patients to steroids as primary therapy for acute graft-versus-host disease: Comparison of grading systems. Biology of Blood and Marrow Transplantation. 2002;**8**(7):387-394. DOI: 10.1053/bbmt.2002.v8.pm12171485

[5] Gooley TA, Chien JW, Pergam SA, Hingorani S, Sorror ML, Boeckh M, et al. Reduced mortality after allogenic hematopoietic-cell transplantation. The New England Journal of Medicine. 2010;**363**:2091-3101. DOI: 10.1056/NEJMoa1004383

[6] Lee SE, Cho BS, Kim JH, Yoon JH, Shin SH, Yahng SA, et al. Risk and prognostic factors for acute GVHD based on NIH consensus criteria. Bone Marrow Transplantation. 2013;**48**:587-592. DOI: 10.1038/bmt.2012.187

[7] Chao NJ. Graft-versus host disease: The view point from the donor T-cell. Biology of Blood and Marrow Transplantation. 1997;**3**:1-10

[8] Martin PJ, Schoch G, Fisher L, Byers V, Anasetti C, Appelbaum FR, et al. A retrospective analysis of therapy for acute graft-versus-host disease: Initial treatment. Blood. 1990;**76**:1464-1472

[9] Sullivan KM, Mori M, Sanders J, Siadak M, Witherspoon RP, Anasetti C, et al. Late complications of allogeneic and autologous marrow transplantation. Bone Marrow Transplantation. 1992;**10**:127-134

[10] Arai S, Arora M, Wang T, et al. Graft-versus-host disease working committee of the CIBMTR. Increasing incidence of chronic graft-versus-host disease in allogeneic transplantation: A report from the Center for International Blood and Marrow Transplant Research. Biology of Blood and Marrow Transplantation. 2015;**21**(2):266-274. DOI: 10.1016/j.bbmt.2014.10.021

[11] Filipovich AH, Weisdorf D, Pavletic S, Socie G, Wingard JR, Lee SJ, et al. National Institutes of Health consensus development project on criteria for clinical trials in chronic graft-versus-host disease: I. Diagnosis and staging working group report. Biology of Blood and Marrow Transplantation. 2005;**11**:945-956

[12] Lee SJ, Klein JP, Barrett AJ, Ringden O, Antin JH, Cahn JY, et al. Severity of chronic graft-versus-host disease: Association with treatment-related mortality and relapse. Blood. 2002;**100**:406-414. DOI: 10.1182/blood.v100.2.406

[13] James LM, Ferrara JLM, Levine JE, Reddy P, Holler E. Graft-versus-host

disease. Lancet. 2009;**373**(9674): 1550-1561. DOI: 10.1016/S0140-6736 (09)60237-3

[14] Bathia S, Francisco L, Carter A, Sun CL, Baker KS, Gurney JG, et al. Late mortality after allogenic hematopoietic cell transplantation and functional status of long-term survivors: Report from the bone marrow transplant survivor study. Blood. 2007;**110**:3784-3792. DOI: 10.1182/blood-2007-03-082933

[15] Billingham RE. The biology of graft-versus-host reactions. Harvey Lectures. 1966-67;**62**:21-78

[16] Aladağ E, Kelkitli E, Göker H. Acute graft-versus-host disease: A brief review. Turkish Journal of Haematology. 2020;**37**(1):1-4. DOI: 10.4274/tjh. galenos.2019.2019.0157

[17] Korngold R, Sprent J. Purified T cell subsets and lethal graft-versus-host disease in mice. In: Gale RP, Champlin R, editors. Progress in Bone Marrow Transplantation. New York: Alan R. Liss; 1987. pp. 213-218

[18] Kernan NA, Collins NH, Juliano LL, Cartagena TT, Dupont BB, OReilly RJ, et al. Lymphocytes in T cell-depleted bone marrow transplants correlate with development of graft-v-host disease. Blood. 1986;**68**:770-773

[19] Jaagia M, Arora M, Flowers ME, Chao NJ, McCarthy PL, Cutler CS, et al. Risk factors for acute GVHD and survival after hematopoietic cell transplantation. Blood. 2012;**119**:296-307. DOI: 10.1182/blood-2011-06-364265

[20] Zeiser R, Blazar BR. Acute graft-versus-host disease biology, prevention and therapy. The New England Journal of Medicine. 2017;**377**(22):2167-2179. DOI: 10.1056/NEJMra1609337

[21] Carapito R, Jung N, Kwemou M, Untrau M, Michel S, Pichot A, et al. Matching for the nonconventional MHC-1 MICA gene significantly reduces the incidence of acute and chronic GVHD. Blood. 2016;**128**:1979-1986. DOI: 10.1182/blood-2016-05-719070

[22] Gooptu M, Koreth J. Translational and clinical advances in acute graft-versus-host disease. Haematologica. 2020;**105**(11):2550-2560. DOI: 10.3324/haematol.2019.240309

[23] Flowers ME, Inamoto Y, Carpenter PA, Lee SJ, Kiem HP, Petersdorf EW, et al. Comparative analysis of risk factors for acute graft-versus-host disease and for chronic graft-versus-host disease according to National Institutes of Health consensus criteria. Blood. 2011;**117**(11):3214-3219. DOI: 10.1182/blood-2010-08-302109

[24] Antin JH, Ferrara JL. Cytokine dysregulation and acute graft-versus-host disease. Blood. 1992;**80**(12):2964-2968

[25] Zeiser R, Blazar BR. Pathophysiology of chronic graft-versus-host disease and therapeutic targets. The New England Journal of Medicine. 2017;**377**:2565-2579. DOI: 10.1056/NEJMra1703472

[26] Soto-Heredero G, Gómez de las Heras MM, Gabandé-Rodríguez F, Oller J, Mittelbrunn M. Glycolisis – A key player in the inflammatory response. The FEBS Journal. 2020;**287**(16):3350-3369. DOI: 10.1111/febs.15327

[27] Palmer CS, Ostrowski M, Balderson B, Christian N, Crowe SM. Glucose metabolism regulates T cell activation, differentiation, and functions. Frontiers in Immunology. 2015;**6**:1. DOI: 10.3389/fimmu.2015.00001

[28] Nguyen H, Haarberg KMK, Wu Y, Fu J, Heinrichs JL, Bastian D,

et al. Allogenic T cells utilize glycolysis as the predominant metabolic pathway to induce acute graft-versus-host disease. Blood. 2014;**124**(21):2419-2419. DOI: 10.1182/blood.V124.212419.2419

[29] Adams WC, Chen YH, Kratchmarov R, Yen B, Nish SA, Lin WHW, et al. Anabolism-associated mitochondrial stasis driving lymphocyte differentiation over self-renewal. Cell Reports. 2016;**17**(12):3142-3152. DOI: 10.1016/celrep.2016.11-065

[30] Beezhold K, Moore N, Chiarannunt P, Brown R, Byersdorfer CA. Deletion of AMP-activated protein kinase (AMPK) in donor T cells protects against graft-versus-host disease through control of regulatory T cell expansion and target organ infiltration. Blood. 2016;**128**(22):806-806. DOI: 10.1182/blood.V128.22.806.806

[31] Gómez-De León A, López-Mora YA, García-Zarate V, Valera-Constantino A, Villegas-De León SU, González-Leal XJ, et al. Impacto f payment source, referral site, and place of residence on outcomes after allogenic transplantation in Mexico. World Journal of Transplantation. 2024;**14**(2):91052. DOI: 10.5500/wjt.v14.i2.91052

Primary and Secondary Prevention: Health Education, Health Promotion, and Specific Protection

Ana Elisa J. Nieto, Mónica Natalia Morales García,
María José Vázquez Reynoso, Carlos García Tapia
and Aarón Humberto Ramírez Mora

Abstract

Graft-versus-host disease (GVHD) is a serious immune complication after an allogeneic hematopoietic stem cell transplant, where donor cells attack the recipient's tissues, mainly affecting the skin, gastrointestinal tract, and liver. It is classified as acute (aGVHD), occurring within 100 days post-transplant, or chronic (cGVHD), which appears later with autoimmune-like symptoms. Risk factors include human leukocyte antigen (HLA) mismatch, advanced recipient age, donor sex, and the intensity of the pre-transplant regimen. Prevention strategies involve genetic testing, careful donor selection, and immunosuppressive therapy with calcineurin inhibitors and corticosteroids. Interdisciplinary management, including specialists such as hematologists, dermatologists, and nutritionists, is crucial for secondary prevention. Early detection of symptoms like rashes, jaundice, and severe diarrhea allows timely intervention to reduce organ damage. Patient education improves treatment adherence and quality of life. Preventive measures such as vaccination, infection control, and optimized immunosuppression help reduce GVHD severity. New research focuses on gut microbiome modulation, cellular therapies, and biomarkers to predict disease progression. These approaches aim to enhance survival and reduce long-term complications in transplant recipients.

Keywords: acute GVHD, chronic GVHD, health education, pre-transplant vaccination, immunosuppressive therapy, infection prevention, antimicrobial prophylaxis

1. Introduction

Graft-versus-host disease (GVHD) is a complex clinical syndrome arising as a major complication that can result after an allogeneic hematopoietic stem cell transplant. When immunocompetent donor cells recognize the recipient's tissues as foreign, they attack them; skin, liver, and gastrointestinal (GI) tract are often affected [1].

We can classify GVHD in two main forms considering its natural course: Acute Graft-Versus-Host-Disease (aGVHD) presents itself during the first 100 days post-transplant with maculopapular rash, nausea, abdominal pain, and profuse diarrhea. As for chronic Graft-Versus-Host-Disease (cGVHD) develops after 100 days and involves multiple organs with autoimmune disease-like symptoms and signs. Various risk factors influence its progression, including human leukocyte antigen (HLA) mismatches between donor and recipient, advanced recipient age, donor gender (particularly in multiparous female donors), the intensity of the pre-transplant conditioning regimen, and source of stem cells (peripheral blood) [1, 2].

2. Primary prevention - Health education and health promotion

2.1 Basic concepts, types, and risk factors

As mentioned before, GVHD is an immune-mediated complication that may occur after an allogeneic stem cell transplant, characterized by a donor T-cell immune response against recipient tissues. Acute and chronic GVHD show separate clinical and temporal characteristics [1].

aGVHD: It mainly affects the skin, liver, and GI tract; symptoms include maculo-papular rash, which may progress to more severe lesions; liver dysfunction, marked by elevated serum bilirubin levels; and GI symptoms such as nausea, vomiting, abdominal pain, and profuse diarrhea. Its severity is graded from I to IV based on the extent and severity of organ involvement.

cGVHD: Although it is described as an entity that develops 100 days post-transplant, its onset may vary. Unlike aGVHD, it can affect almost any organ and mimics systemic autoimmune diseases, such as scleroderma and lichen planus. Ocular involvement frequently manifests as dry eye syndrome. Other symptoms include dry mouth, liver dysfunction, obstructive lung disease, and GI involvement. Chronic GVHD is classified as mild, moderate, or severe, depending on the extent of organ involvement and its impact on the patient's quality of life. The most commonly affected organs, in descending order, are the skin, mouth, liver, eyes, intestines, lungs, vagina, esophagus, joints, nails, muscles, and serosa [1, 2].

Traditionally, acute and chronic GVHD were distinguished by their onset before or after 100 days post-transplant. However, they are now categorized depending on distinct pathophysiological mechanisms and clinical presentation. In the early stages, inflammatory changes prevail due to alloimmune reactivity. Over time, autoimmune and immunodeficiency processes lead to tissue damage through fibrosis and repair mechanisms. Although GVHD follows a dynamic and overlapping course, not all patients develop both forms, as they emerge from different pathophysiological mechanisms and are studied separately. According to the latter, the National Health Institutes classifies the disease as classic aGVHD; persistent, recurrent, or late-onset aGVHD; classic cGVHD, and overlap syndrome [2].

2.1.1 Risk factors

Several factors increase the risk of developing GVHD, including HLA disparity between donor and recipient, advanced age of both, and donor gender, particularly when a female donates to a male recipient. Additionally, the use of peripheral blood stem cells instead of bone marrow and the intensity of the pre-transplant conditioning regimen can influence GVHD incidence and severity [1, 3].

2.2 Patient and family education

Education and preparing patients and their families or support networks is essential for improving clinical outcomes and quality of life. They must understand the associated risks and the possibility of developing GVHD. This also allows early recognition of symptoms, leading to timely intervention and reduced morbidity; treatment adherence and active participation in the recovery process are related to this education as well [4].

Early detection of GVHD is critical for effective management. The onset can be insidious, with symptoms often being mild and overlooked by the patient until significant organ damage occurs. Patients and caregivers should be aware of the following symptoms:

Skin: Rashes, redness, or peeling.

Gastrointestinal tract: Persistent diarrhea, nausea, vomiting, or abdominal pain.

Liver: Jaundice (yellowing of the skin and eyes), dark urine, or abdominal swelling.

Eyes: Dry eyes or excessive tearing.

Structured educational programs with patient-oriented informative sessions might be helpful for patients and families. Educational pamphlets have proven to be effective too, as patients can keep them as reminders or tools for monitoring their condition [5].

2.3 Nutrition and lifestyle

A multidisciplinary approach is essential for these patients. Proper nutrition and a healthy lifestyle are critical for minimizing the risk of GVHD and improving the quality of life for affected patients [6].

A balanced diet is key to strengthening the immune system and promoting post-transplant recovery. A diet rich in proteins, vitamins, and minerals, including fresh fruits and vegetables, whole grains, and lean protein sources, is recommended. It is crucial to avoid foods that may be contaminated or difficult to digest, such as raw or undercooked foods, to reduce the risk of infections. In some cases, a bland, lactose-free diet may be suggested to aid digestion and minimize gastrointestinal discomfort [7, 8].

2.3.1 Infection control

Bacterial, viral, or fungal infections in post-transplant patients require focused attention, especially in those at high risk for or diagnosed with GVHD. Strict hygiene measures, such as frequent handwashing and surface disinfection, must be followed. Additionally, avoiding contact with sick individuals and crowded places, such as hospitals or healthcare centers, is advised to reduce exposure to pathogens [9].

2.3.2 Healthy habits

Maintaining healthy habits contributes to faster recovery and better quality of life. Moderate physical exercise, tailored to the patient's capabilities, is recommended to improve blood circulation and strengthen the cardiovascular system. It is also essential to maintain proper hydration and avoid harmful substances, such as alcohol and tobacco, which can impair immune function and increase the risk of infections or other complications [1, 7].

2.4 Emotional and psychological support

In addition to conventional medical treatments, emotional and psychological support plays a crucial role in managing graft-versus-host disease (GVHD), as stress and negative emotions can influence the patient's immune response.

2.4.1 Stress reduction strategies

Adopting stress management techniques is essential for patients with GVHD. Practices such as meditation, deep breathing, and mindfulness have proven effective in reducing anxiety and improving overall well-being. These techniques help patients focus on the present moment, decreasing worry about the future and promoting relaxation [10].

Additionally, engaging in activities that promote relaxation, such as therapeutic music, can have a positive impact on mood and stress reduction. For example, the foundation Musicians for Health has implemented micro-concerts in hospitals, demonstrating that music can enhance the well-being of both patients and healthcare professionals [11].

2.4.2 Impact on immunity

Chronic stress can negatively affect the immune system, increasing susceptibility to infections and complications. Therefore, effective stress management not only improves emotional well-being but also has direct benefits for the patient's physical health. Reducing stress contributes to better immune function, which is vital for the recovery and management of GVHD.

2.4.3 Caregiver support

It is important to recognize that caregivers of patients with GVHD also face significant emotional challenges. Providing them with psychological support and self-care strategies is essential for their well-being and the quality of care they offer. Support programs and educational resources can help caregivers manage the stress and emotions associated with caring for a loved one with GVHD [12].

2.4.4 Treatment adherence

The multidisciplinary approach, which includes psychological support, also influences treatment adherence, such as taking immunosuppressive medications and following other prophylactic measures. It is crucial that patients strictly follow medical instructions regarding dosing and administration schedules to ensure the treatment's effectiveness. Non-adherence can increase the risk of disease development and compromise therapy outcomes. Patients must understand the importance of following medical recommendations and maintain constant communication with their healthcare team to address any concerns and adjust treatments as necessary [13, 14].

2.5 Pre-transplant vaccination

For vaccination in patients undergoing allogeneic hematopoietic stem cell transplantation, the state of immunosuppression, the impact of immunosuppressive treatments, and the risk of graft-versus-host disease (GVHD) relapse must be evaluated. Regarding the patient's condition, vaccination is delayed until immune reconstitution is achieved, which varies from 6 to 12 months post-transplant. However, if active acute GVHD or immunosuppressive use is present, vaccination may be further postponed. In the case of active chronic GVHD or GVHD dependent on immunosuppression, vaccination is modified based on the patient's stability [15].

Vaccines that are recommended include inactivated vaccines, administered according to the recommended schedule. For example, the influenza vaccine is recommended annually during the winter season. Additionally, conjugate vaccines against pneumococcus (PCV13) and polysaccharide vaccines (PPSV23), the *Haemophilus influenzae* type B (Hib) vaccine, the hepatitis B (HBV) vaccine, tetanus, diphtheria, and whooping cough vaccines (Tdap or Td), and the meningococcal ACWY and B vaccines for patients at risk are also recommended [15, 16]. Live attenuated vaccines, such as the measles, mumps, and rubella (MMR) vaccine and the varicella vaccine, are contraindicated due to the high risk of disseminated infection from the vaccine strain. These vaccines can be administered in patients with controlled GVHD, without immunosuppression, and at least 24 months after transplantation [17].

The vaccination schedule should be individualized based on the patient's characteristics and the recommendations of the country, considering local incidence.

A typical schedule begins between 6 and 12 months post-transplant (if there is no active GVHD):

- 6–12 months: Influenza, PCV13, Hib, hepatitis B, Tdap.

- 12–24 months: PPSV23, meningococcus, hepatitis A (if necessary).

- 24+ months (without active immunosuppression): MMR and varicella, if indicated [18].

Genetic Counseling and Pre-transplant Testing: Identifying Potential Incompatibilities to Prevent Graft-versus-Host Disease (GVHD).

Genetic counseling and pre-transplant testing are crucial for preventing graft-versus-host disease (GVHD), transplant success, and reducing complications. The success of the transplant depends largely on the compatibility between the donor and recipient, as well as the evaluation of genetic and immunological factors [19].

2.6 Key aspects of genetic counseling and pre-transplant testing

2.6.1 HLA typing (human leukocyte antigen)

- The most critical component for selecting compatible donors. It includes:

  o HLA-A, HLA-B, HLA-C (Class I)

  o HLA-DRB1, HLA-DQB1 (Class II)

- An identical HLA match (10/10) is required for both related and unrelated allogeneic transplants.

- HLA mismatches can increase the risk of GVHD and graft failure [20].

2.6.2 Evaluation of minor histocompatibility alleles

These are recognized by the immune system and can trigger GVHD.

2.6.3 Additional immunogenetic testing

- Hematopoietic chimerism: Determines the presence of donor and recipient cells post-transplant. Useful for assessing the likelihood of rejection or GVHD.

- KIR typing (Killer Immunoglobulin-like Receptors): Evaluates NK cell immune receptors.

- Genetic polymorphisms: Factors like IL-10, TNF-α, and other inflammation-related genes can influence the severity of GVHD.

2.6.4 Evaluation of anti-HLA antibodies

Patients may develop anti-HLA antibodies through previous transfusions, pregnancies, or transplants. The presence of these antibodies is associated with an increased risk of rejection and GVHD.

2.6.5 Genetic counseling for underlying diseases

Identifying genetic mutations associated with hereditary hematological diseases can influence patient preparation for transplantation [19, 20].

2.6.6 Strategies for preventing GVHD with pre-transplant testing

- Rigorous donor selection:

  Prefer HLA-identical related donors.
  Consider umbilical cord stem cell banks if no compatible donor is available.

- Pre-transplant conditioning:

  Adjust the conditioning regimen based on the immunological risk identified in genetic testing.

- Post-transplant immunoprophylaxis:

  Reduce the immune response of the graft with agents such as cyclosporine, tacrolimus, methotrexate, cyclophosphamide, or antithymocyte globulin [21].

2.7 Immunity and infection prevention

Patients undergoing transplantation often have a compromised immune system due to their underlying disease and prior treatments, such as chemotherapy and radiation therapy.

2.7.1 Pre-transplant care to strengthen immunity

Pre-transplant Vaccination: The goal is to protect the patient against preventable infections during immunosuppression.
Recommended vaccines:

- Influenza (inactivated virus)

- Pneumococcus (PCV13 and PPSV23)

- Hepatitis B

- *Haemophilus influenzae* type B (Hib)

- Tetanus, diphtheria, and whooping cough (Tdap)

- Meningococcus (ACWY and B, if necessary)

- Live attenuated vaccines (e.g., measles and varicella) should be administered at least 4 weeks before starting the conditioning regimen.

2.7.2 Treatment of active infections

Identify and treat any active infections before the transplant (bacterial, viral, fungal, and parasitic infections).
Diagnostic tests are recommended to determine the source of infection:

- Blood cultures, urine cultures, and secretion cultures.

- Serologies for latent viruses like CMV, EBV, HBV, HCV, and HIV.

- Tuberculosis tests.

- Evaluation for fungal diseases, such as galactomannan in at-risk patients.

2.7.3 Antimicrobial prophylaxis

Initiate prophylaxis based on the patient's risk:

- Bacterial: Fluoroquinolones in patients with prolonged neutropenia.

- Fungal: Azoles (fluconazole and voriconazole) in patients at high risk for fungal infections. Trimethoprim-sulfamethoxazole to prevent *Pneumocystis jirovecii*.

- Viral: Acyclovir or valacyclovir in seropositive patients for herpes simplex or varicella-zoster.

2.7.4 Nutritional assessment

Improving nutritional status is crucial since malnutrition compromises immunity. A diet rich in proteins, vitamins (A, C, D, and E), and minerals (zinc and selenium) is recommended, along with supplementation if deficiencies are present.

2.7.5 Oral care

Reduces the risk of oral infections that could complicate the transplant. It is essential to treat cavities, gingivitis, or abscesses before the procedure.

2.7.6 Reducing exposure to pathogens

Frequent handwashing, wearing masks in high-risk environments, and avoiding contact with sick individuals.

2.7.7 Latent infection assessment

Viral reactivations are common, and identifying latent carriers allows for appropriate prophylaxis or monitoring.

2.7.8 Physical conditioning

Maintain a moderate exercise routine tailored to the patient's tolerance to strengthen the immune system and enhance post-transplant recovery [22, 23].

3. Secondary prevention - Specific protection

3.1 Early identification

3.1.1 Clinical signs

- Acute GVHD:

  o Skin (50–75% of cases):

  o Appears as an erythematous maculopapular rash that starts on palms, soles, and trunk, potentially spreading.

  o Severe desquamation or blister formation.

  o Liver:

  o Elevation of total bilirubin, transaminases, and alkaline phosphatase.

  o Jaundice and hepatomegaly in advanced cases.

  o Gastrointestinal tract:

o Watery diarrhea (>500 ml/day).

o Abdominal pain, nausea, vomiting, and gastrointestinal bleeding.

- Chronic GVHD:

o Skin changes similar to scleroderma.

o Xerostomia and alterations in oral mucosa.

o Dry eye syndrome.

o Obliterative bronchiolitis.

o Progressive liver dysfunction [24].

3.1.2 Diagnostic tests

- Biopsy of affected tissues:

o Gold standard for confirming the diagnosis.

Typical findings: keratinocyte apoptosis in the skin, lymphocytic infiltration in the liver, and crypt atrophy with apoptosis in the intestines.

- Liver evaluation:

o Liver profile: elevated conjugated bilirubin, transaminases, and alkaline phosphatase.

- Imaging tests:

o Endoscopy or colonoscopy.

o Liver ultrasound.

- Tests to exclude other causes:

o Stool cultures to identify pathogens.

o Serological tests and PCR for viral infections [25].

3.1.3 Biomarkers: To detect early stages and predict severity

- Acute GVHD biomarkers:

o ST2 (interleukin-1 signaling suppressor): Elevated in the presence of intestinal damage, indicating higher mortality.

o Reg3α (regenerating islet-derived protein 3-alpha): Indicates intestinal damage.

    o Elafin: Indicates skin damage.

    o Soluble IL-2R (sIL-2R): Elevated in active GVHD due to T-cell activation.

- Chronic GVHD biomarkers:

    o BAFF (B-cell activating factor): Associated with B-cell activation.

    o CXCL9 and CXCL10: Indicators of inflammation [26].

3.2 Adjusted immunosuppressive therapies

Optimizing immunosuppressive therapies in post-transplant patients aims to balance the prevention of graft-versus-host disease (GVHD) with maintaining adequate immune function to prevent infections and other complications. This is achieved through the customization of the immunosuppressive regimen based on factors such as the risk of GVHD, the patient's clinical condition, and the response to treatment.

3.2.1 Principles of immunosuppressive treatment optimization

- Individualization:

Adjustments based on weight, liver and kidney function, and patient tolerance.

- Therapeutic drug monitoring (TDM):

Regular assessment of serum levels to avoid toxicity or therapeutic failure.

- Stepwise strategies:

Use of combinations of low doses of multiple agents to minimize side effects [23, 24].

3.2.2 Common immunosuppressive medications

- Calcineurin inhibitors:

    o Drugs: Cyclosporine and tacrolimus.

    o Mechanism: Block T-cell activation.

    o Optimization:

    o TDM: Cyclosporine serum levels (100–400 ng/mL) and tacrolimus (5–20 ng/mL).

    o Side effects: Nephrotoxicity, hypertension, and diabetes.

- Antimetabolites:

o Drugs: Mycophenolate mofetil (MMF) and methotrexate.

o Mechanism: Inhibit lymphocyte proliferation.

o Optimization:

o Dose adjustment based on renal function.

o Side effects: Myelosuppression, diarrhea.

- Corticosteroids:

o Drug: Prednisone.

o Mechanism: Inhibit inflammatory response and T-cell activation.

o Optimization:

o Short-term use to control acute episodes.

o Gradual reduction to avoid long-term side effects (osteoporosis and hyperglycemia).

- Biological agents:

o Drugs: Antithymocyte globulin (ATG), rituximab, and infliximab.

o Mechanism: Act on specific lymphocytes or inflammatory molecules.

o Optimization:

o Used in severe or refractory cases.

o Monitoring for opportunistic infections.

- mTOR inhibitors:

o Drugs: Sirolimus and everolimus.

o Mechanism: Block IL-2-mediated cell proliferation.

o Optimization:

o Considered as an alternative in cases of nephrotoxicity from calcineurin inhibitors.

o Monitoring of serum levels (5–15 ng/mL).

3.2.3 Adjusting treatment based on risk

- Low-risk GVHD patients: Monotherapy with a calcineurin inhibitor or sirolimus.

- High-risk GVHD patients: Combination therapy with a calcineurin inhibitor, mycophenolate, and corticosteroids.

- ATG prophylaxis in some cases.

- Acute GVHD:

  Mild to moderate: Increase corticosteroids (2 mg/kg/day of prednisone).

  Severe: Inclusion of biological agents (infliximab or ruxolitinib).

- Chronic GVHD:

  Substitute corticosteroids with mTOR inhibitors or rituximab to minimize long-term toxicity.

3.2.4 Emerging strategies

- Cyclophosphamide

- Targeted Therapies:

  JAK inhibitors (e.g., ruxolitinib) for refractory cases.

- Cellular Therapies:

  Use of regulatory T-cells (Tregs) to modulate the immune response.

- Predictive Biomarkers:

  Incorporating biomarkers (ST2 and Reg3α) to personalize dosing [26, 27].

3.3 Antimicrobial prophylaxis

Antimicrobial prophylaxis, including the use of antibiotics, antivirals, and anti-fungals, is essential in the secondary prevention of GVHD, as infections can trigger or worsen the disease.

3.3.1 Antibiotics

Prophylactic administration of broad-spectrum antibiotics is common in post-transplant patients to prevent bacterial infections. However, it is crucial to adjust the antibiotic regimen based on the patient's microbiota and the local prevalence of resistant pathogens. The indiscriminate use of antibiotics can lead to the selection of resistant microorganisms, complicating the management of future infections.

3.3.2 Antivirals

Antiviral prophylaxis is key to preventing infections by viruses such as cytomega-lovirus (CMV), which can be reactivated in immunocompromised patients. The use of antiviral medications, such as valganciclovir, is recommended for patients at high risk of viral reactivation. Regular monitoring of viral load is essential to adjust therapy and prevent CMV reactivation, which can trigger or worsen GVHD.

3.3.3 Antifungals

Antifungal prophylaxis is necessary to prevent fungal infections, especially in patients with prolonged neutropenia. The use of broad-spectrum antifungals, such as posaconazole, is recommended for patients at high risk of invasive fungal infections. Monitoring of liver and kidney function is essential during antifungal therapy to prevent adverse effects and adjust dosing as needed [28].

3.4 Post-transplant immunization

Post-transplant immunization is essential for maintaining adequate protection against infections, as the immunosuppressive regimen used to prevent GVHD can compromise the patient's immune response.

3.4.1 Considerations for post-transplant immunization

3.4.1.1 Evaluation of the patient's immunological status

Before starting any vaccination regimen, it is crucial to assess the patient's immune function, considering factors such as the type of transplant, the intensity of the conditioning regimen, and the time elapsed since the transplant.

3.4.1.2 Vaccination schedule

It is recommended to begin immunization with inactivated vaccines at least 6 months after the transplant, once the immune function has stabilized. Live attenuated vaccines should be avoided during the first 2 years post-transplant due to the risk of associated illness.

3.4.1.3 Recommended vaccines

The recommended inactivated vaccines include influenza, pneumococcal, hepatitis B, tetanus-diphtheria-acellular pertussis (Tdap), and herpes zoster vaccines. Pneumococcal vaccination is especially important, as post-transplant patients are at higher risk for pneumococcal infections.

3.4.1.4 Monitoring the immunological response

It is essential to evaluate the response to vaccines by measuring antibody titers. In case of an insufficient response, additional doses or the use of specific immunoglobulins can be considered.

3.4.1.5 Patient education and follow-up

Patient education on the importance of immunization and regular follow-up are crucial to ensure adequate protection against infections [28, 29].

3.5 Dermatological and gastrointestinal care

Target organ involvement, such as the skin and gastrointestinal tract, is common in graft-versus-host disease (GVHD). Secondary prevention, focusing on the specific protection of these organs, is essential for improving outcomes in post-transplant patients.

3.5.1 Dermatological care

The skin is one of the primary organs affected by GVHD. Preventing skin lesions and protecting against infections are critical. The use of emollients is recommended to maintain skin hydration and prevent dryness. Additionally, it is crucial to avoid exposure to the sun and excessive heat, as the skin of post-transplant patients is more susceptible to damage. Regular skin monitoring allows for the early detection of lesions and timely intervention.

3.5.2 Gastrointestinal care

The gastrointestinal tract is also a target organ in GVHD. Preventing gastrointestinal infections and managing symptoms such as diarrhea are essential. A balanced and appropriate diet is recommended, avoiding foods that may irritate the digestive tract. Proper hydration is crucial to prevent dehydration associated with diarrhea. Additionally, monitoring gastrointestinal signs and symptoms is important for early intervention.

Implementing specific measures for the protection of the skin and gastrointestinal tract is essential in the secondary prevention of GVHD. Comprehensive care, including appropriate dermatological and gastrointestinal management, along with constant monitoring, can significantly improve the quality of life and outcomes in post-transplant patients [30].

3.6 Early therapeutic interventions: Strategies to limit disease progression when detected early

The implementation of early therapeutic interventions is essential in the secondary prevention of GVHD, aiming to minimize the incidence and severity of the disease.

3.6.1 Early intervention strategies

3.6.1.1 Pharmacological prophylaxis

The administration of immunosuppressive agents, such as tacrolimus and methotrexate, has been established as an effective strategy to prevent GVHD. These medications inhibit the activation and proliferation of T-cells from the graft, reducing the immune response against the host. Recent studies have shown that these prophylactic regimens are equally effective in preventing GVHD, although overall survival may be slightly lower in patients receiving T-cell depletion.

3.6.1.2 T-cell depletion

The removal of T-cells from the graft before transplantation may reduce the incidence of GVHD. However, this strategy may be associated with lower overall survival compared to other prophylactic regimens.

3.6.1.3 Gut microbiome modulation

Recent research suggests that manipulating the gut microbiome could influence the incidence of GVHD. Ongoing studies are investigating whether increasing intestinal bacterial diversity can reduce the risk of developing GVHD.

3.6.1.4 Cellular and gene therapies

Therapies that modulate the immune response by manipulating T-cells or genetically modifying them are being investigated, with the goal of preventing GVHD without compromising graft efficacy.

3.6.2 Importance of early intervention

Early identification and treatment of GVHD are crucial for improving outcomes in post-transplant patients. The implementation of therapeutic strategies from the early post-transplant stages can reduce the morbidity and mortality associated with GVHD.

Early therapeutic interventions are critical in the secondary prevention of GVHD. A combination of pharmacological prophylaxis, T-cell depletion, gut microbiome modulation, and cellular therapies provides a comprehensive approach to minimize the incidence and severity of GVHD, thereby improving the quality of life and long-term outcomes for transplant recipients.

3.7 Interdisciplinary support

The implementation of an interdisciplinary healthcare team is essential in the secondary prevention of GVHD, as it enables comprehensive and personalized patient care.

GVHD affects multiple organ systems, including the skin, gastrointestinal tract, and liver. A diverse healthcare team, composed of hematologists, immunologists, dermatologists, gastroenterologists, nutritionists, and psychologists, among others, is crucial for addressing the various manifestations of the disease and its complications [7, 31].

3.7.1 Key roles of the interdisciplinary team

3.7.1.1 Evaluation and diagnosis

Each specialist contributes their expertise to a thorough evaluation of the patient, enabling accurate and early diagnosis of GVHD.

3.7.1.2 Therapeutic planning

Collaboration among professionals allows for the design of a personalized treatment plan that considers the individual characteristics of each patient and the specific manifestations of GVHD.

3.7.1.3 Monitoring and follow-up

Constant monitoring of patients is essential to detect complications early and adjust treatment as needed.

3.7.1.4 Emotional and psychological support

GVHD can significantly impact the patient's quality of life. Psychological support is crucial to help the patient and their family cope with the emotional challenges associated with the disease and treatment [32].

4. Conclusion

Both primary and secondary prevention require a multidisciplinary team since this is key in preventive aspects as well as the follow-up of the patient and the family in order to achieve a greater quality of life and treatment adherence, hence lower morbidity and mortality.

Acknowledgements

The authors declare that they used AI tools (ChatGPT) to enhance translation from Spanish to English.

Author details

Ana Elisa J. Nieto[1]*, Mónica Natalia Morales García[1], María José Vázquez Reynoso[1], Carlos García Tapia[2] and Aarón Humberto Ramírez Mora[1]

1 General Hospital of Leon, Institute of Public Health of the State of Guanajuato, Mexico

2 Regional High Specialty Hospital of Bajío, Leon, Guanajuato, Mexico

*Address all correspondence to: anaelisajnieto@gmail.com

IntechOpen

References

[1] Flowers MED, Vogelsang GB. Clinical manifestations and natural history. In: Chronic Graft Versus Host Disease. Cambridge University Press; 2009. pp. 56-69

[2] Enfermedad injerto contra huésped [Internet]. Available from: www.LLS.org/espanol

[3] Choo SY, The HLA. System: Genetics, immunology, clinical testing, and clinical implications. Yonsei Medical Journal. 2007;**48**(1):11

[4] Cuvelier GDE, Schoettler M, Buxbaum NP, Pinal-Fernandez I, Schmalzing M, Distler JHW, et al. Toward a better understanding of the atypical features of chronic graft-versus-host disease: A report from the 2020 National Institutes of Health consensus project task force. Transplantation and Cellular Therapy. 2022;**28**(8):426-445

[5] Penack O, Marchetti M, Aljurf M, Arat M, Bonifazi F, Duarte RF, et al. Prophylaxis and management of graft-versus-host disease after stem-cell transplantation for haematological malignancies: Updated consensus recommendations of the European Society for Blood and Marrow Transplantation. Lancet Haematology. 2024;**11**(2):e147-e159

[6] Jagasia MH, Greinix HT, Arora M, Williams KM, Wolff D, Cowen EW, et al. National Institutes of Health consensus development project on criteria for clinical trials in chronic graft-versus-host disease: I. The 2014 diagnosis and staging working group report. Biology of Blood and Marrow Transplantation. 2015;**21**(3):389-401.e1

[7] van der Meij BS, de Graaf P, Wierdsma NJ, Langius JAE, Janssen JJWM, van Leeuwen PAM, et al. Nutritional support in patients with GVHD of the digestive tract: State of the art. Bone Marrow Transplantation. 2013;**48**(4):474-482

[8] Limpert R, Pan P, Wang LS, Chen X. From support to therapy: Rethinking the role of nutrition in acute graft-versus-host disease. Frontiers in Immunology. 2023;**14**

[9] Pereira AZ, Gonçalves SEA, Rodrigues M, Hamerschlak N, Flowers ME. Challenging and practical aspects of nutrition in chronic graft-versus-host disease. Biology of Blood and Marrow Transplantation. 2020;**26**(11):e265-e270

[10] Blood & Marrow Transplant Information Network. Coping with stress caused by graft-versus-host disease. BMT InfoNet [Internet]. [citado 2025 Feb 5]. Disponible en: https://bmtinfonet.org/transplant-article/coping-stress-gvhd

[11] Bradt J, Dileo C, Magill L, et al. Music interventions for improving psychological and physical outcomes in cancer patients. Cochrane Database of Systematic Reviews. 2016;(8):CD006911. Available from: https://www.cochranelibrary.com

[12] Michelle Bishop P. ¡Los Cuidadores de Paciente de Enfermedades de Injerto contra Huésped también son Sobrevivientes! 2023;10

[13] Rotz SJ, Bhatt NS, Hamilton BK, Duncan C, Aljurf M, Atsuta Y, et al. International recommendations for screening and preventative practices for long-term survivors of transplantation and cellular therapy: A 2023 update. Transplantation and Cellular Therapy. 2024;**30**(4):349-385

[14] Bolaños-Meade J, Hamadani M, Wu J, Al Malki MM, Martens MJ, Runaas L, et al. Post-transplantation cyclophosphamide-based graft-versus-host disease prophylaxis. New England Journal of Medicine. 2023;**388**(25):2338-2348

[15] Hilgendorf I, Freund M, Jilg W, Einsele H, Gea-Banacloche J, Greinix H, et al. Vaccination of allogeneic haematopoietic stem cell transplant recipients: Report from the international consensus conference on clinical practice in chronic GVHD. Vaccine. 2011;**29**(16):2825-2833

[16] Rubin LG, Levin MJ, Ljungman P, Davies EG, Avery R, Tomblyn M, et al. Executive summary: 2013 IDSA clinical practice guideline for vaccination of the immunocompromised host. Clinical Infectious Diseases. 2014;**58**(3):309-318

[17] Cordonnier C, Einarsdottir S, Cesaro S, Di Blasi R, Mikulska M, Rieger C, et al. Vaccination of haemopoietic stem cell transplant recipients: Guidelines of the 2017 European conference on infections in leukaemia (ECIL 7). The Lancet Infectious Diseases. 2019;**19**(6):e200-e212

[18] Ljungman P, Cordonnier C, Einsele H, Englund J, Machado CM, Storek J, et al. Vaccination of hematopoietic cell transplant recipients. Bone Marrow Transplantation. 2009;**44**(8):521-526

[19] Socié G, Ritz J. Current issues in chronic graft-versus-host disease. Blood. 2014;**124**(3):374-384

[20] Carreras E, Dufour C, Mohty M, Kröger N, editors. The EBMT Handbook. Cham: Springer International Publishing; 2019

[21] Bray RA, Hurley CK, Kamani NR, Woolfrey A, Müller C, Spellman S, et al. National marrow donor program HLA matching guidelines for unrelated adult donor hematopoietic cell transplants. Biology of Blood and Marrow Transplantation. 2008;**14**:45-53

[22] Sullivan KM, Dykewicz CA, Longworth DL, Boeckh M, Baden LR, Rubin RH, et al. Preventing opportunistic infections after hematopoietic stem cell transplantation: The Centers for Disease Control and Prevention, Infectious Diseases Society of America, and American Society for Blood and Marrow Transplantation Practice Guidelines and beyond. Hematology. 2001;**2001**(1):392-421

[23] Tomblyn M, Chiller T, Einsele H, Gress R, Sepkowitz K, Storek J, et al. Guidelines for preventing infectious complications among hematopoietic cell transplantation recipients: A global perspective. Biology of Blood and Marrow Transplantation. 2009;**15**(10):1143-1238

[24] Zeiser R, Blazar BR. Pathophysiology of chronic graft-versus-host disease and therapeutic targets. New England Journal of Medicine. 2017;**377**(26):2565-2579

[25] Levine JE, Logan BR, Wu J, Alousi AM, Bolaños-Meade J, Ferrara JLM, et al. Acute graft-versus-host disease biomarkers measured during therapy can predict treatment outcomes: A blood and marrow transplant clinical trials network study. Blood. 2012;**119**(16):3854-3860

[26] Hill GR, Ferrara JLM. The primacy of the gastrointestinal tract as a target organ of acute graft-versus-host disease: Rationale for the use of cytokine shields in allogeneic bone marrow transplantation. Blood. 2000;**95**(9):2754-2759

[27] Martin PJ, Rizzo JD, Wingard JR, Ballen K, Curtin PT, Cutler C, et al. First- and second-line systemic treatment of acute graft-versus-host disease: Recommendations of the American Society of Blood and Marrow Transplantation. Biology of Blood and Marrow Transplantation. 2012;**18**(8):1150-1163

[28] Lee TH, Huang CT, Lin CC, Chung CS, Lin CK, Tsai KC. Similar rebleeding rate in 3-day and 7-day intravenous ceftriaxone prophylaxis for patients with acute variceal bleeding. Journal of the Formosan Medical Association. 2016;**115**(7):547-552

[29] L'Huillier AG, Kumar D. Immunizations in solid organ and hematopoeitic stem cell transplant patients: A comprehensive review. Human Vaccine Immunotherapeutics. 2015;**11**(12):2852-2863

[30] Gomez-Venegas AA, Mosquera-Klinger G, Carvajal Gutiérrez JJ, Juliao Baños F, Goldstein Rothstein A, Pérez Cadavid JC, et al. Compromiso gastrointestinal por enfermedad de injerto contra huésped. Revista Colombiana de Gastroenterología. 2022;**37**(2):225-232

[31] Naymagon S, Naymagon L, Wong SY, Ko HM, Renteria A, Levine J, et al. Acute graft-versus-host disease of the gut: Considerations for the gastroenterologist. Nature Reviews. Gastroenterology & Hepatology. 2017;**14**(12):711-726

[32] Marcela C, Cancino H, Petersen RC, Nemoto I, Sasada V, Dillenburg CS, et al. Enfermedad injerto contra huésped: Sus manifestaciones bucales graft-versus-host disease: Its oral manifestations [Internet]. Revista Cubana de Estomatología. 2017;**54**. Available from: http://scielo.sld.cu

Chapter 3

Pathogenic Period: Clinical Stage of Graft-Versus-Host-Disease

Fanny Guadalupe López-Gómez,
Roberto Francisco Vázquez-Caballero
and Neylly Benítez-Muñoz

Abstract

Graft-versus-host disease, in its acute and chronic presentation, is one of the pathologies that require timely diagnosis since it is one of the most common causes of morbidity and mortality associated with hematopoietic stem cell transplantation when it is performed on patients who, due to some medical situation, require a transplant, receiving a graft by chimerism. In this case, chimerism originates through the transplant of an organ or bone marrow from another person (donor). This condition can occur because the recipient has organs from two genetically different living beings, so some cells or tissues in a person's body contain at least two types of DNA. The timeliness of diagnosis is directly related to the early identification of signs and symptoms, so this chapter reviews the clinical manifestations of graft vs. host disease with the purpose of providing specific treatment in a timely manner. In the acute form, it manifests with skin changes such as maculopapular rash and jaundice and is accompanied by diarrhea. In the chronic form, it generally affects multiple organs, manifesting in the skin, eyes, mouth, lungs, genitals, gastrointestinal tract, and musculoskeletal system. An additional review of the differences between acute and chronic forms of host versus graft disease is carried out.

Keywords: graft versus host disease, early diagnosis, symptoms, signs, acute GVHD, chronic GVHD

1. Introduction

Hematopoietic stem cell transplantation (HSCT) is a therapy used to treat high-risk malignant hematologic disorders and other life-threatening hematologic and genetic diseases [1].

Graft-versus-host disease (GVHD) is the main complication of allogeneic hematopoietic stem cell transplantation and organs containing lymphoid cells. Considered a major complication of allogeneic hematopoietic cell transplantation, it occurs when the immune cells of the graft donor become sensitized and attack the host tissues [2].

It is a multisystem disease and is based on the recognition of the recipient's tissues by the donor's inherited immunity.

It has two forms of presentation, acute and chronic, with particular clinical, immunological, and histological characteristics depending on its pathophysiology and clinical presentation [3, 4].

2. Clinical data

The initial designation of GVHD was proposed by Billingham in 1966 [5], who stated the following criteria for the presentation of this entity: the graft must contain immunologically competent cells, the recipient must express tissue antigens that are not present in the transplant donor, and the patient must be unable to generate an effective response to eliminate the transplanted cells.

2.1 Acute GVHD

In acute disease occurring within 3 months after transplantation [6], the appearance of maculopapular rash, jaundice, and diarrhea is characterized. While in chronic disease, it tends to affect multiple organs and is characterized by involvement of the skin, eyes, mouth, lungs, genitals, gastrointestinal tract, and musculoskeletal system [2].

According to the American Society for Blood and Marrow Transplantation (ASBMT), the acute form is classified as classic when it occurs before 100 days posttransplant or in the context of a donor lymphocyte infusion (DLI) and may present with maculopapular rash, nausea, vomiting, anorexia, diarrhea, ileus, and cholestatic hepatitis; the persistent, recurrent, or late-onset acute occurs after 100 days posttransplant or a DLI. It presents the clinical characteristics of classic acute GVHD without diagnostic or distinctive manifestations of chronic GVHD (**Table 1**) [6].

2.1.1 Cutaneous manifestations

Erythematous papular rash, which may be asymptomatic, pruritic, or painful. This occurs between days 7 and 21 post-transplant, mainly affecting the palms and soles. It then spreads to the earlobes, cheeks, neck, and trunk, and from there, it can

Grade	Skin	Liver	Gastrointestinal	Functional impairment
0 (None)	0	0	0	0
I (Mild)	1–2	0	0	0
II (Moderate)	1–3	1	1	1
III (Severe)	2–3	2–3	2–3	2
IV (Threat to life)	2–4	2–4	2–4	3

Each grade is based on the highest stage for each organ involved.
Each column identifies the lowest stage for each organ.
Grade IV may also include lesser organ involvement but with a large decrease on the functional rating scale [7].

Table 1.
Clinical grades of aGVHD according to Seattle's criteria.

merge and involve the entire skin. The rash may be scarlatiniform, with subsequent peeling and evolution with hyperpigmented areas.

There is a hyperacute variant that is very rare; it occurs between the first and the second week post-transplant and includes fever, rapid progression of the rash with epidermal detachment, blistering lesions, a positive Nikolsky sign, and involvement of mucous membranes.

This variant resembles toxic epidermal necrolysis and is the most severe form of acute cutaneous GVHD [6–9].

2.1.2 Gastrointestinal manifestations

Nausea, vomiting, diarrhea when there is decreased intestinal absorption, abdominal pain, and ileus may indicate severe involvement.

Liver involvement manifests with increased transaminases (TGP) and direct bilirubin, hepatomegaly, and jaundice [8, 9].

2.2 Chronic GVHD

The chronic GVHD (cGVHD) is similar to autoimmune diseases such as scleroderma; histologically, there is a marked increase in collagen deposition and fibrosis in the affected organs, associated with a high production of autoantibodies. Donor T cells recognize specific host antigens in the skin and blood that trigger alloreactivity and autoreactivity phenomena. The appearance of hemolytic anemia, thrombocytopenia, anti-lymphocyte antibodies, and autoantibodies against the nucleus, nucleolus, smooth muscle, thyroid, and skin has been demonstrated [10].

2.2.1 Classification of cGVHD according to the ASBMT

Classic chronic: This is the type of GVHD that, regardless of the time of onset, does not present characteristics of acute GVHD [2, 11, 12]. It presents with manifestations that can be attributed solely to cGVHD [2]. Its manifestations on the skin are: poikiloderma, lichen planus-like lesions, scleroderma, morphea-like, and lichen sclerosis-like lesions. In the mouth: lichen-like lesions, hyperkeratotic plaques, or restriction of mouth opening due to sclerosis).

Overlap syndrome: Presentation with distinctive manifestations of chronic disease, along with typical characteristics of acute disease: presence of 1 or more symptoms of acute disease in a patient diagnosed with chronic disease; the manifestations may be present during the initial diagnosis of a chronic disease or may arise after the initial diagnosis; and acute symptoms may recur regardless of whether chronic manifestations resolve or persist [2].

The cGVHD can be limited or extensive. The cutaneous manifestations can be in two categories: Early-onset lichenoid lesions.

Early-onset lichenoid lesions are characterized by erythematous-violaceous papules or plaques with superficial adherent desquamation that sometimes merge, compromising large areas. The affected areas are the periorbital area, ears, palms, and soles, and it may affect nails, causing onychoatrophy and nail loss. At the genital level, it may cause phimosis or vaginal constriction. It may cause fibrosis in the joints, causing contractures [8, 9, 11].

Late-onset scleroderma lesions. The disseminated scleroderma form may present as guttate or confetti-like, as plaques of morphea without a liliaceous ring located

Organs	Signs	Symptoms
Skin Nails Hair	Lichen planus, lichen sclerosis, inability to sweat, ichthyosis, keratosis pilaris, hypopigmentation, hyperpigmentation, erythema, poikiloderma, maculopapular rash, nail dystrophy, Ptengion unguis Alopecia depigmentation of hair, Papulosquamous lesions on the scalp	Itching, dryness, nail detachment, thinning hair, premature graying
Vulvovaginal	Lichen planus, vaginal stenosis, erosions, fissures, ulcers	Dyspareunia, vaginal dryness
Muscles, fascia, joints	Fasciitis, sclerosis, myositis, or polymyositis, edema	Joint numbness, muscle cramps, arthralgia or arthritis, weakness
Eyes	Scarring conjunctivitis, Keratoconjunctivitis, sicca punctate keratopathy, blepharitis	Dryness, tearing, or pain in the eyes Photophobia
Gastrointestinal tract	Esophageal stricture, pancreatic insufficiency, vomiting, diarrhea	Anorexia, nausea, weight loss, failure to thrive, abdominal cramps
Liver	Hyperbilirubinemia transaminasemia	Jaundice
Lung	Bronchiolitis obliterans	dyspnea
Hematopoiesis - immune system	Anemia, thrombocytopenia, eosinophilia, hyper or hypogammaglobulinemia, Autoantibodies (AIHA, PTI)	
Other	Peripheral neuropathy, nephrotic syndrome, myasthenia gravis, abnormalities in the cardiac conduction system, cardiomyopathy, coronary fibrosis.	Specific symptoms of each pathology

Source: Own design based in [11].

Table 2.
Clinical data of cGVHD [11].

on the trunk and in the proximal region of the limbs, buttocks, and thighs. The skin appendages may present areas of alopecia, nail dystrophy, decreased sweating, and decreased secretion of the tear and salivary glands, giving rise to a picture similar to sicca (Sjögren's syndrome), there may also be Acro sclerosis and Raynaud's phenomenon (**Table 2**) [8, 9, 11].

2.2.2 Ocular manifestations

Less than 10% of aGVHD patients suffer ocular involvement, which manifests as pseudomembranous conjunctivitis and corneal involvement [13].

Ocular involvement is associated with an increased risk of death [14], and ocular involvement is found in 30–85% of cGVHD cases, and although ocular manifestations generally occur after other alterations, they can occasionally be the debut of aGVHD [15].

3. Conclusions

Knowledge of the symptoms of GVHD for its diagnosis remains the fundamental pillar for supportive treatment, so it is important to consider that comprehensive and continuous monitoring must be provided *to* identify and treat any type of complication that may arise in an accurate manner and thus preserve the patient's life.

aGVHD, in turn, is classified as mild, moderate, or severe, depending on the affected organs.

It can occur in the first 3 months of life (+7 to +21 days). The main symptoms are dermatological alterations such as erythematous papular rash and scarlatiform rash. In this same context, we should not fail to consider a rare form called hyperacute, in which there is a rash with epidermal detachment (blistering lesions).

Other extracutaneous lesions are of the gastrointestinal tract, such as nausea, vomiting, diarrhea, and liver disease that manifests with increased bilirubin and glutamic pyruvic transaminase (GPT).

In the review of this *chapter*, we conclude that cGVHD (Chronic Graft-versus-Host Disease) is the most severe form of this entity. We can detect it after +21 days after the graft, taking into account that its presentation is similar to that of some autoimmune diseases such as scleroderma and that it can simultaneously affect several organs.

Therefore, if it is detected in its acute or initial phase, we can prevent multi-organ involvement and improve the quality of life of patients, and consequently, the high costs in the treatment and management of complications could be reduced.

Conflict of interest

The authors declare no conflict of interest.

Author details

Fanny Guadalupe López-Gómez[1]*, Roberto Francisco Vázquez-Caballero[2] and Neylly Benítez-Muñoz[2]

1 Pediatrics Department, Hospital General San Luis de la Paz, Institute of Public Health from Guanajuato State, San Luis de la Paz, México

2 Teaching Department, Hospital General San Luis de la Paz, Institute of Public Health from Guanajuato State, San Luis de la Paz, México

*Address all correspondence to: fanny.pediatra@gmail.com

IntechOpen

References

[1] Ferrara JLM, Levine JE, Reddy P, Holler E. Graft-versus-host disease. Lancet. 2009;**373**(9674):1550-1561. DOI: 10.1016/s0140-6736(09)60237-3

[2] Kurya AU, Aliyu U, Tudu AI, Usman AG, Yusuf M, Gupta S, et al. Graft-versus-host disease: Therapeutic prospects of improving the long-term post-transplant outcomes. Transplantation Reports. 2022;**7**(4): 100107. DOI: 10.1016/j.tpr.2022.100107

[3] Ballester-Sánchez R, Navarro-Mira M, Sanz-Caballer J, Botella-Estrada R. Aproximación a la enfermedad injerto contra huésped cutánea. Actas Dermo-Sifiliográficas. 2016;**107**(3):183-193. DOI: 10.1016/j.ad.2015.10.003

[4] Velasquez MM. Enfermedad injerto contra huésped. Rev. Asoc. Colomb. Alerg. Inmunol. 2001;**10**(4):110-118. Available from: https://pesquisa.bvsalud. org/portal/resource/pt/lil-346693

[5] Billingham RE. The biology of graft-versus-host reactions. Harvey Lectures. 1966-67;**62**:21-78

[6] Kliegman RM. Nelson Textbook of Pediatrics. 22st ed. Vol. 2. Philadelphia: Elsevier; 2025. pp. 1356-1360

[7] Stringa MF. Enfermedad de injerto contra huésped cutánea en el trasplante alogénico de médula ósea. Dermatología Argentina. 2010;**16**(4):252-261. Available from: https://www.dermatolarg.org.ar/ index.php/dermatolarg/article/view/497

[8] Molés PP, Botella ER, Sanz BJ. La Fe IIS. Caracterización Clínica, Histológica y Biológica de la Enfermedad de Injerto Contra Huésped Cutánea Aguda y Crónica. Tesis doctoral. Valencia: IIS La Fe;

2024. Available from: https://www. iislafe.es/es/sociedad/eventos/461/ caracterizacion-clinica-histologica-y biologica-de-la-enfermedad-de-injerto-contra-huesped-cutanea-aguda-y-cronica

[9] Cardoza T, Ocampo-Candiani J. Enfermedad injerto contra huésped y sus manifestaciones cutáneas. Medicina Cutánea Ibero-Latino-Americana. 2011;**39**(3):95-105. Available from: https://www.medigraphic.com/cgi-bin/ new/resumen.cgi?IDARTICULO=31503

[10] Jaime Fagundo JC, Dorticós Balea E, Pavón Morán V, Jauma Rojo AJ, Cortina RL. Aspectos inmunológicos del trasplante de células progenitoras hematopoyéticas. Revista cubana de hematología, immunología y hemoterapia. 2006;**22**(3):0-0. Available from: http://scielo.sld.cu/scielo. php?script=sci_arttext&pid=S0864-02892006000300003&lng=es

[11] López-Hernández G, Olaya-Vargas A, Pérez-García M, Mora-Magaña I. Pronóstico de la enfermedad de injerto contra huésped aguda y crónica en pacientes pediátricos sometidosa trasplante de precursores de células hematopoyéticas. Experiencia del programa de trasplante de células progenitoras hematopoyéticas en el Instituto Nacional de Pediatría. Tesis para obtener el Diploma de AltaEspecialidad Médica. Universidad Nacional Autónoma de México. 2012. Available from: http:// repositorio.pediatria.gob.mx:8180/ handle/20.500.12103/3102

[12] Lasierra Viguri L, García Gil A, García Gil FA. Enfermedad del injerto contra el huésped en trasplante de hígado. Revisión de literatura. Trabajo de Fin de Grado. Departamento de Cirugía, Ginecología y Obstetricia,

Área de Cirugía, Zaguan, Repositorio
Institucional de Documentos,
Universidad de Zaragoza, Med; 2016.
Available from: https://zaguan.unizar.es/
record/57509

[13] Soleimani M, Sharif PM,
Cheraqpour K, Koganti R, Masoumi A,
Baharnoori SM, et al. Ocular graft-
versus-host disease (oGVHD): From
a to Z. Survey of Ophthalmology.
2023;**68**(4):697-712. DOI: 10.1016/j.
survophthal.2023.02.006

[14] Saito T, Shinagawa K, Takenaka K,
et al. Ocular manifestation of acute
graft-versus-host disease after
allogeneic peripheral blood stem cell
transplantation. International Journal of
Hematology. 2002;**75**:332-334

[15] Shikari H, Amparo H, Saboo U,
Dana R. Onset of ocular graft-after
allogenic hematopoietic stem cell
transplantation. Cornea. 2015;**34**:243-247

Chapter 4

Second-Line Treatment of aGvHD: State of the Art and Novel Therapies

Abdellatif Bouazzaoui

Abstract

Allogeneic stem cell transplantation (alloSCT) is a unique curative therapy for diverse hematological and malignant diseases. However, after alloSCT, more than 50% of the patients develop acute and/or chronic graft-versus-host disease (a/cGvHD), which remains the major cause of mortality and morbidities with high impact on the life quality. Corticosteroids are considered as the first-line therapy; a complete response occurs in 25–40% of the patients. But a prolonged application of the steroid results in steroid-resistant in about 40% of patients and also in different complications. These make the development of new agents as second-line treatment for aGVHD of high importance. In this chapter, we will describe the characteristics and manifestations of aGvHD, and we will discuss the currently known second-line treatments including extracorporeal photopheresis (ECP) and different immunosuppressive drugs like antithymocyte globulin, alemtuzumab, (mTOR) kinase inhibitors, anti-tumor necrosis factor (TNF)-α antibodies, anti-IL-2 receptor antibodies, and others. Furthermore, we will discuss the recent advances in cell therapies like the use of decidua stromal cells (DSCs), mesenchymal stromal cells, and microbiome and give in addition an overview of treatment costs.

Keywords: stem cell transplantation, graft-versus-host disease, bioactive compounds, mesenchymal stromal cells, decidua stromal cells

1. Introduction

Allogeneic stem cell transplantation (allo-HSCT) using hematopoietic stem cells from a donor is a vital treatment for many diseases such as nonmalignant, hematologic malignancies, and cancer diseases [1]. Every year, the number of bone marrow transplants to patients increases. In 2022, more than 46,143 HSCT (41.2% allogeneic and 58.8% autologous) were reported by 689 European centers [2]. HSCT is considered as successful solution in treating diseases, but it leads also to serious complications, such as graft-versus-host disease (GVHD). These are the result of an attack by the donor's immune cells against the recipient's tissues and is considered one of the fatal complications resulting from HSCT [3–5]. GVHD disease can occur at any time after HSCT and can appear in two forms, aGVHD or cGVHD. Both forms are classified based on time of onset after HSCT and the criteria from the NIH 2014 for cGVHD [6, 7] and Mount Sinai Acute GVHD International Consortium (MAGIC) for aGVHD [8]. The latter form of GVHD appears in 30–50% of patients who received HSCT from matched related donors. Furthermore, in the USA during 2017–2018 and among the recipients from closely matched related persons, 13% of recipients died due to complications of GVHD within or after 100 days of receiving HSCT [9]. Corticosteroid therapy is considered one of the primary and most important treatments against GVHD; however, it remains ineffective in a significant number of cases, ranging from 30 to 50% of the persons received stem cell transplantation. Cases that do not respond to corticosteroids or steroid refractory GVHD (SR-GVHD) have a poor prognosis (6 months at around 50%). In this context, identifying the causes and mechanisms that lead to SR-GVHD and the development of new treatments for people who suffer from SR-GVHD in order to increase survival is very critical and urgent.

2. Manifestation and characteristics of aGVHD and cGVHD

After transplantation allo-HSCT from matched related donors, approximately 50% of the patients could develop aGVHD [4, 10–13]. In typical cases, the aGVHD develops within 100 days after blood transfusion. But in some cases, it can appear after 100 days. The disease appears as an acute inflammatory condition affecting the gastrointestinal (GI) tract, skin, and liver. But there are more of evidences that the aGVHD may affect other target organs including the nervous system, kidneys, thymus, testis, ovaries, and bone marrow [14, 15]. The aGVHD is clinically classified from first to fourth grade according to the extent of skin involvement, liver, and GI tract [8]. The manifestation for the GI aGVHD can be divided into upper manifestations such as vomiting, nausea, and anorexia and lower GI manifestation including hematochezia, ileus, diarrhea, and abdominal cramping and pain. The severity of the GI aGVHD can be determined by the volume of diarrhea that can continue even after abstain from eating. In the case of skin aGVHD, the patient develops a rash on the shoulders, around the neck, soles of the feet, the hands, and the eyes [4]. The severity of the skin aGVHD can be determined by the area of skin affected.

In patients who have received allo-HSCT from matched related donors, cGVHD is considered as the leading cause of late death [16, 17]. The number of patients diagnosed with the cGVHD after allo-HSCT may reach up to 70%, and the most patients develop cGVHD symptoms between 100 and 1 years after receiving allo-HSCT, whereas around 10% of the patients showed the symptoms later. The important thing to mention is that some patients develop the cGVHD without showing any prior signs of acute illness [18–21]. The manifestations and symptoms of the disease are multiple and varied, as it may begin with inflammation in different organs resulting in fibrosis and organ failure [21–23].

3. First-line treatment against aGVHD

Since the aGVHD is the result of an acute inflammatory condition, it is necessary that the treatment inhibits this reaction. Glucocorticoids (GCs) are very effective against various autoimmune/inflammatory diseases such inflammatory bowel disease, asthma, rheumatoid arthritis, and others [24–30]. Furthermore, GCs are also used in organ transplantation and hematological malignancies [31, 32]. In this context, a systemic application of a strong dose of corticosteroids is considered the best option [33]. Patients with aGVHD grade II to IV are injected with a steroid dose ranging from 1 to 2 mg/kg [33–36] to reduce the inflammation and is considered for long time as the first-line treatment against aGVHD [37–43]. However, the use of high-dose of GCs for long time has also several side effects, including opportunistic infections [10] diabetes, alteration of behavior, muscle atrophy, skin disorders, and fat dysregulation [32, 44]. In addition, about 40% of patients with aGVHD do not respond to treatment with GCs and develop SR-aGVHD [45] which can appear 3–5 days if the patients showed in clear significant improvement and 5–10 days if there is no improvement [46]. For 50% of the patients with SR-aGVHD, their survival period does not exceed 6 months, and less than 30% of the SR-aGVHD patients have a survival for more than 2 years [13, 35, 47, 48]. Taking all of the above, it becomes clear that understanding the mechanisms causing the SR-aGVHD represents a very urgent and pressing need to develop new treatments against the SR-aGVHD to save the lives of patients with aGVHD.

4. Second-line treatment against aGVHD

In case, the use of steroids does not give any effect, the SR-aGVHD appears. At that time the question is what is the treatment should be followed? Until now, there is no ideal treatment nor a standard protocol for care and treatment against SR-aGVHD [45, 49–51], but there are multiple treatment options such as the use of antibodies, including anti–IL-2 receptor antibodies, anti-tumor necrosis factor (TNF)-a antibodies, anti-CD3/CD7, anti-CD25, and anti-CD26. Other treatment options are the use of extracorporeal photopheresis (ECP), mammalian target of rapamycin (mTOR) inhibitors (sirolimus or everolimus), antithymocyte globulin (ATG), mycophenolate mofetil, etanercept, alemtuzumab, and others [35, 45, 46, 50]. Furthermore, there are new methods based on microbiome, cell therapies such as mesenchymal stromal cells (MSC) and decidua stromal cells (DSCs) as cells therapy which showed promising results.

5. JAK1 and JAK2 kinase inhibitor

Among the second-line treatments against SR-aGVHD, we find ruxolitinib among the most documented drug [52], and ruxolitinib is a Janus kinase (JAK) 1/JAK2 inhibitor, which influences pathogenesis of aGvHD significantly [53]. On May 24, 2019 ruxolitinib has been approved by the FDA as second-line treatment for patients with SR-aGVHD based on a multicenter, open-label phase 2 trial study (REACH-1, NCT02953678) [54]. In this study, patients aged 12 years and older received initially a twice-daily dose of 5 mg, which was increased to 10 mg over 3 days. The median survival (MS) reached 7.6 months, the overall response rate (ORR) was 73.2%, and 56.3% of the patients showed a complete response (CR). Later, on Sep. 22, 2021, the FDA has also approved the ruxolitinib for the treatment of cGVHD, based on the results evaluated in REACH-3 (NCT03112603) study, a randomized, open-label, multicenter trial [55]. In this study, 165 patients received 10 mg of the ruxolitinib twice a day and were compared to 164 patients how received best available therapy (BAT). The study finds that the median duration of response was 4.2 months for the ruxolitinib versus 2.1 months for the BAT patients. In a previous REACH-2 study from the same author [52], 154 patients were treated with ruxolitinib and were compared with 155 patients in the control group. The authors find that ruxolitinib was effective, but it was accompanied by toxic symptoms such as thrombocytopenia.

Another drug used in the treatment of aGVHD is itacitinib, and this is a JAK1-inhibitor with efficacy in preclinical study. In the study, Schroeder et al. used 200 mg or 300 mg itacitinib daily to treat 29 patients with SR-aGVHD [56]. The ORR on day 28 reached 75 and 66.7%, respectively, and the overall survival (OS) was 58.6 and 48.3% at 6 and 12 months. Recently, in a double-blind, phase 3 international clinical trial (GRAVITAS-301), Zeiser et al. study the effect of itacitinib (NCT03139604) [57]. In this study, the patients received steroids/itacitinib (n = 219) or steroids/placebo (n = 220). At day 28, the authors find that the ORR reached 74% for itacitinib and 66% for placebo, and the improvement did not reach a significant level, which makes it necessary to conduct in-depth research to investigate the selective JAK1 inhibition of itacitinib.

5.1 Antibodies and antagonists

5.1.1 Anti-CD3/CD7immunotoxin (CD3/CD7-IT)

As treatment for patients with SR-aGVHD, CD3/CD7 immunotoxin (CD3/CD7-IT) is an anti-CD3/CD7 mixture conjugated ricin which was given in a phase I/II trial study including 20 patients [58]. The study showed that an ORR of 60% at day 28 with 50% of the patients reached a CR. The author finds also that the treatment at early stage caused profound depletion of T cells and NK cells.

5.1.2 Inolimomab

Inolimomab is an anti-CD25 monoclonal antibody used in the treatment of patients with SR-aGVHD. The treatment with inolimomab blocks the interleukin-2 receptor α (IL-2Rα), and it showed encouraging results based on a randomized, multicenter, open-label, phase III trial (EUDRACT 2007-005009-24), which was conducted by Gérard Socié et al. [59]. In this study, 100 patients with SR-aGVHD received treatment with inolimomab (n = 49) or ATG (n = 51). The author finds a survival of 28.5% in the inolimomab group versus 21.5% in the ATG group. Side effects were similar in both groups, with more viral infections in inolimomab patients. In the follow-up period after 1 year, the author reached a survival of 47% in the inolimomab group and 40% in the ATG patients [60].

5.1.3 Infliximab

The proinflammatory cytokine including TNF is highly expressed in GVHD [61], and Infliximab, a TNF-alpha inhibitor, is considered as a good treatment for patients with SR-aGVHD. In this context, Couriel et al. analyzed the effect of infliximab in a prospective, single-center, open label, randomized, phase III study, and in this study, 63 patients with SR-aGVHD received infliximab plus methylprednisolone or methylprednisolone alone (control). At day 28, the ORR reached 62% in infliximab group versus 58% in the control group. Non-relapse mortality (NRM) and OS were not significantly different [62]. In a recent retrospective study from Nygaard et al., the author treated 68 patients (grade III-IV) with infliximab, and the response was analyzed at day 7 and 28 after treatment. The author finds that 60% of the patients (n = 41) respond at day 7, whereas 46% (n = 31) respond at day 28. Patients with response to infliximab have higher OS probability than non-responders [63].

5.1.4 Etanercept

Another TNF blocker is etanercept, a recombinant human-soluble TNF receptor fusion protein. In a study conducted by Busca et al., 21 patients with SR-GVHD (13 aGVHD and 8 cGVHD) were treated with etanercept. The results showed that 52% (n = 11) of the patients respond to the treatment (6 patients with aGVHD and 5 with cGVHD). The CR and PR were 5 (4 with aGVHD and 1 with cGVHD) and 6 (2 with aGVHD and 4 with cGVHD), respectively. Furthermore, the result showed that 67% of the patients (n = 14) were alive after a median follow-up of 429 days [64].

5.1.5 Alemtuzumab

Alemtuzumab is an antibody against the CD52 antigen, and all cells expressing this antigen such as B lymphocytes natural killer, dendritic cells, and monocytes will be a target for alemtuzumab. In a prospective study conducted by Khandelwal et al., fifteen patients with SR-aGVHD (grad II-IV) received alemtuzumab. The ORR was 67%, CR in 40%, 27% with PR, and no response in 33% [65]. The most important side effects appeared are asymptomatic viremias (100%), transient thrombocytopenia (53%), and fever (26%). After 6 months, 80% of patients were alive (n = 12).

5.1.6 Daclizumab

Daclizumab is an antagonist against IL-2Rα, and in a prospective, single-center, phase II study, Bordigoni et al. treated 62 patients with daclizumab as single second-line treatment [66]. The results showed a CR in 68.8% of the patients, and the 4-year event-free survival (EFS) reached 54.6%. In a previous study conducted by Soltani et al., the author finds that treatment of SR-aGVHD patients with daclizumab in combination with infliximab (TNF blocker) showed a better probability to achieve a CR with long-term survival of 40% [67].

5.1.7 Basiliximab

Basiliximab is also another antibody to target the IL-2Rα. In one recent study recruited patients from 36 hospitals, Basiliximab was used as single (n = 642) or in combination with other treatments (n = 298), the study showed an ORR of 79.4% at day 28, the OS 3 years after treatment reached 64.3%, and probabilities of NRM were 26.8% [68].

5.1.8 Vedolizumab

Vedolizumab is an antibody against the integrin subunit alpha 4beta 7 (α4β7 integrin) which is expressed on the surface of the lymphocytes. The application of vedolizumab inhibits the interaction between α4β7 integrin and mucosal addressing cellular adhesion molecule1 (MAdCAM-1) and stops the lymphocytes relocation to the GI tract [69]. In a recent study from Chen et al. conducted during the

COVID-19 pandemic, the author treated 168 patients with vedolizumab or placebo (n = 165), and the results showed 70.9% GI aGVHD-free survival at day 180 after transplantation versus 70.9% for placebo patients [70]. In an early prospective study conducted by Mehta et al., the author treated 20 patients with gastrointestinal SR-aGVHD with vedolizumab. After 59 days, the results showed CR and ORR of 20 and 25%, respectively. The most side effects were infections and liver enzymes elevation [71].

5.1.9 Begelomab

Begelomab is an anti-CD26 antibody, and the CD26 is considered as potential target for the treatment of aGVHD because it has a costimulatory function and is expressed on the activated T-cells. In study from Bacigalupo et al., the author treated 28 patients with SR-aGVHD in two prospective studies and 41 patients in one compassionate study. In the prospective studies, the results showed that the ORR, CR, and one-year OS reached 75%, 11%, and 50%, respectively, whereas the ORR was 61%, the CR reached 12%, and the one-year OS was 30% in the compassionate study. However, the patients developed few side effects such as bronchopneumonia, *E. coli* infection, bacterial sepsis, renal failure, acute respiratory failure, multiorgan failure, convulsions, and dyspnea [72]. In a previous study and based on the data collected from 110 patients, the NRM in control at day 180 reached 50% versus 25% in begelomab [73], and the OS at 1 year was 31% in control versus 50% in patients treated with begelomab.

5.1.10 Visilizumab

Visilizumab is an antibody against CD3 that induces a selective apoptosis in activated T-cells. In a multicenter phase II study, Carpenter et al. used visilizumab to treat 44 patients with SR-aGVHD and grade III or IV acute GVHD. At day 42, the ORR and CR reached 32% and 14%, respectively, and the OS at 180 days reached 32% [74]. Beside GVHD as main reason for die, further reasons were multiorgan failure, infection, recurrent malignancy, hemorrhagic pancreatitis, fatal arrhythmia, and myocardial infarction. In a previous study, 11 patients with SR-aGVHD received a single dose of 3.0 mg/m^2 on day 1. The results showed that 6 patients have CR, 3 patients with partial response (PR), and 7 patients have a MS of 359 days (260–490 days) [75].

5.2 Alpha-1 antitrypsin (AAT)

During the GVHD, proinflammatory cytokines are significantly increased, in preclinical study. The application of AAT, a serine protease antiapoptotic, anti-inflammatory and immunomodulatory properties resulted in lower expression of different proinflammatory cytokines such as tumor necrosis factor (TNF), IL-1 and IL-32 [76]. In a phaseI/II single-center study, the author treated 12 patients with SR-aGVHD (grad III-IV) intravenously. The treatment resulted in significant improvement in 8 patients, with 4 patients have CR, and 50% were a live at last follow-up [77]. In the previous phase 2 clinical trial study (NCT01700036), patients with SR-aGVHD were treated with AAT [78]. At day 28, the results showed 65% of ORR and the CR of 35%. Furthermore, the response maintains at 73% after 60 days. Interestingly, the infection mortality maintains at 10% after 6 months and within 30 days only 2.5%.

5.3 mTOR inhibitor

Sirolimus and everolimus are mTOR inhibitors used as second-line treatment against SR-aGVHD. In a pilot study from Benito et al., 21 patients (GVHD grad III-IV) not responding to steroid were treated with sirolimus [79]. The first group received a loading dose (15 mg/m^2) on day 1 followed by 5 mg/m^2/day, and the other 2 groups received or 4 mg/m^2/day or 5 mg/m^2/day sirolimus for 14 days without a loading dose. The results of the study showed that the treatment with sirolimus has activity against SR-aGVHD, the ORR was 57%, and the CR reached 24%. However, this effect was accompanied by a high toxicity, and this confirms the need for further studies to determine the appropriate dose. Sirolimus was also used as control in the REACH2 trial study from Zeiser et al. [52]. In a recent retrospective study conducted by Biavasco et al., another mTOR inhibitor (everolimus) has been used in 6.5% of the patients as control and was compared to ruxolitinib [80].

5.4 Nucleoside inhibitor

Pentostatin an adenosine deaminase inhibitor is also used as treatment against SR-aGVHD. In a phase I study, 23 patients were treated intravenously with a dose escalation of pentastatin starting with 1 mg/m^2/day. The result showed that 63% of the patients reached CR, 14% PR and the MS was 85 days. The study also showed that the treatment was well tolerated with a slight increase in thrombocytopenia and liver function tests [81].

6. Other adjunct therapy

In addition to the treatments mentioned above, there are also auxiliary treatments used to treat aGVHD. These include hormone therapy such as the human chorionic gonadotropin (HCG), extracorporeal photopheresis (ECP) therapy, cell therapy including mesenchymal stromal cells (MSCs) and decidua stromal cells (DSCs), and finally the treatment of aGVHD using microbiota.

6.1 HCG therapy

Hormone therapy, such as HCG, is a new method used to treat aGVHD. This hormone has the ability to increase the level of the epidermal growth factor (EGF) in the blood circulation which leads to accelerating the process of tissue regeneration. Due to the commercial availability and easy accessibility of HCG, it has been used as a treatment in the previous studies. In a recent open-label prospective phase II clinical trial (NCT02525029), G Holtan et al. study the effect of HCG as treatment against aGVHD. In the study, 22 patients with grade III-IV aGVHD or stage 3–4 lower GI-GVHD received methylprednisolone and urine-derived HCG (uHCG). At day 28 after treatment, the results of the study find that 68% of the patients showed a response (57% with CR, 11% with PR) [82]. In a previous study used HCG as therapy for SR-aGVHD, the results showed 60% response (CR or PR) [83, 84].

6.2 Extracorporeal photopheresis (ECP)

This method uses ultraviolet rays to destroy the white blood cells that cause aGVHD. Since 1988, the ECP has been approved by the FDA as treatment against the leukemic cutaneous T-cell lymphoma [85]. After that on 1990, the method was used in the treatment of aGVHD. During the ECP, the mononuclear cells were isolated, exposed to UV irradiation in combination with 8-methoxypsoralen and reinfusion. Recently, in a randomized controlled trial study from Maryan M Ali et al., 157 patients (between 18 and 74 years) were randomized, 76 patients were treated with ECP, and 81 patients as the control group. The per-protocol analysis showed a significant difference in GVHD between the control group (n = 77) versus intervention group, and the values reached 68 versus 46%, respectively [86]. However, the NRM, OS, GVHD-free, relapse-free survival, and event-free survival did not differ significantly.

6.3 Cell therapy against aGVHD

Cell therapy including MSCs is considered one of the new methods of treatment against GVHD. Furthermore and in contrast to pharmacological immunosuppressive drugs, in the use of cell therapy, the long-term side effects are absent, while the side effects and toxicity are very few and may be non-existent [87, 88].

6.3.1 Mesenchymal stromal cells (MSCs)

A group of cells like MSCs and, to a lesser extent, T_{reg} cells are used as a treatment for a group of diseases including SR-aGVHD [89]. One of the advantages of MSCs is their ability to produce and transform into a group of specialized cells such as hepatocytes. Osteocytes, adipocytes, chondrocytes, and neurocytes [90]. One of the advantages of MSCs is that they can be easily isolated at low cost from several tissues, including, but not limited to adipose tissue placenta, umbilical cord, and amniotic membrane. MSCs have emerged as a treatment for several types of diseases, including GVHD [91–93]. In addition to the ability of MSCs to renew a group of cells, they cause minimal immune response due to the lack of HLA class-II and costimulatory molecules on its cell membrane. The MSCs also acquire an anti-inflammatory property and immunosuppressive activity [94–96]. The first case in which the feasibility of stem cells in treating GVHD was studied in Sweden (Karolinska Institute) [97]. After that, in 2008, Le Blanc et al. published results using MSCs therapy. In the study, 55 patients with SR-GVHD were treated with MSCs, and after 1 year after the infusion, the results showed that 30 patients had a CR and nine showed PR. The most importantly, the study proved that the infusion with MSCs does not cause any side effects [98]. After that, several studies were conducted worldwide to study the effect of MSCs in treating GVHD [87, 91, 92, 99–101]. There are also several countries including Korea, Japan, Canada, and New Zealand that have licensed MSCs products as a treatment against aGVHD [102, 103]. Among these products, we find Remestemcel-L (Ryoncil™, Mesoblast, Ltd), which was well tolerated and did not cause any side effects or toxicities or other safety concerns. Recently, FDA approved Remestemcel-L as treatment for SR-aGVHD based on the results collected from a phase 3, single-arm, prospective multicenter study (NCT02336230) [104]. In this study, Kurtzberg et al. have showed the efficacity of MSCs against aGVHD in 54 children with primary SR-aGVHD.

6.3.2 Decidua stromal cells (DSCs)

The DSCs derived from the placenta are stromal cells with origin from the mother. The decidua is a uterine tissue playing an important role in maternal-fetal immune tolerance [105, 106]. Several studies have proven that DSCs differ from MSCs in several aspects, including, but not limited to its ability to cause more effective clotting compared to MSCs. DSCs are also able to inhibit the proliferation of T cells whether they are frozen and thawed or fresh [107–114]. Regarding the use of DSCs as a treatment for SR-aGVHD, different studies have been shown to be effective in improving the outcome. In a long-term follow-up of a pilot study from Sadeghi et al., 21 patients with grade II-IV GVHD were treated with DSCs. The results showed that 11 patients have a CR and 10 patients with PR. Furthermore, the cumulative incidence of cGVHD reached 52%, and the OS was 57% [115]. In a phase I/II trial study from Ringdén and Sadeghi, the author treated 21 patients with DSCs, and the median cell dose was 1.2×10^6 cells/kg body weight. The results showed that all patients responded, with CR in 11 patients, PR in 10 patients, and the1-year survival reached 81% [116].

6.4 Microbiota

Several recent studies have proven the important role of microbiota, especially those colonizing the intestines, in influencing a group of diseases, including GVHD. A few recently published studies have shown that feces can be transferred to the recipient without any complication, and it is safe and effective as treatment against GVHD [117]. In a recent publication from Qiao et al., the author used meta-analysis data to study the effect of fecal microbiota transplantation (FMT) as treatment for patients with SR-aGVHD [118]. In this study, data from 23 studies with a total of 242 patients were included. The meta-analysis study showed that 100 patients reached CR and 61 patients achieved PR, whereas 81 patients not responded. The most side effect caused by the FMT was infection (3 patients), but the patients recovered after treatment. Based on these results, FMT is considered as good alternative for the treatment of SR-aGVHD. In another phase II trial study from Rashidi et al., the patients received oral encapsulated, third-party FMT and were compared with placebo patients. At day 180 after FMT, the results showed at day 180 that the incidence of grade II–IV aGVHD was reduced in the group with more donor microbiota fraction (dMf) [119]. The author concluded that fecal transfusion leads to an improvement in the condition of patients, especially those who have a significant change in the intestinal microbiota. In a randomized, double-blind placebo-controlled trial (NCT06026371), Reddi et al. tested if the transfer of healthy-donor FMT early after alloHCT reduces the incidence and severity of aGVHD or not. In the study, 20 patients received FMT from three different healthy donors. The results showed that the microbiota engraftment rate from the third donor was higher compared to the first and second donors and reaching 66%. These results prove the necessity of selecting the appropriate donor to achieve good results.

7. Costs for therapies against aGVHD

The costs for the second and adjunct therapies are generally quite expensive, especially when the patient is exposed to complications. This limits the ability to treat a large number of patients. The average cost of ECP treatment is up to $9000 ($500–$100,000) [120]. Regarding stem cell therapy, the cost ranges between $1200 and $28,000 [121]. For the TNF blockers, the costs vary between $14,000 and $25,000 (Etanercept the lowest and infliximab the highest) [122]. For the mTOR inhibitor the monthly costs are between $1000 and $2000 [123], and for the IL-2Rα, the costs are around $3000 per basiliximab dose [124]. The dose for ATG costs also $3000 [124].

The treatment with JAK inhibitor such as ruxolitinib is also quite expensive, and it costs about $83,000 for 6 months [123]. Tyrosin Kinase inhibitor like belumosudil is also expensive, and for 1 year, it can reach $232,000 [125]. The only exception regarding the prices is represented by uHCG, because this medicine is commercially available and therefore inexpensive, the cost per vial reaches $296 [126].

8. Conclusion

HSCT is a very effective treatment for several types of hematological malignancies and other fatal disorders. Since decades, corticosteroid therapy is considered one of the primary and most important treatments against GVHD; however, it remains ineffective in a up to 50%. Cases with SR-GVHD have a poor prognosis. For this reason, there is an urgent need to discover other treatments as a second line of defense. There are several treatments, including drug therapy, cell therapy, and microbiome therapy. But it still suffers from several drawbacks, the most important of which are the very high prices, there is no ideal treatment nor a standard protocol for using the treatment. This requires more effort and work to overcome it.

Conflict of interest

The authors declare no conflict of interest.

Author details

Abdellatif Bouazzaoui
Department of Internal Medicin III (Haematology and Internal Oncology), University Hospital Regensburg, Franz-Josef-Strauß-Allee, Regensburg, Germany

*Address all correspondence to: ab1971@hotmail.de

IntechOpen

References

[1] Granot N, Storb R. History of hematopoietic cell transplantation: Challenges and progress. Haematologica. 2020;**105**(12):2716-2729

[2] Passweg JR, Baldomero H, Ciceri F, de la Cámara R, Glass B, Greco R, et al. Hematopoietic cell transplantation and cellular therapies in Europe 2022. CAR-T activity continues to grow; transplant activity has slowed: A report from the EBMT. Journal of Bone Marrow Transplantation. 2024;**59**(6):803-812

[3] Jagasia M, Zeiser R, Arbushites M, Delaite P, Gadbaw B, Bubnoff NV. Ruxolitinib for the treatment of patients with steroid-refractory GVHD: An introduction to the REACH trials. Journal of Immunotherapy. 2018;**10**(5):391-402

[4] Ferrara JL, Levine JE, Reddy P, Holler E. Graft-versus-host disease. Lancet. 2009;**373**(9674):1550-1561

[5] Zeiser R, Negrin RS. Introduction to a review series on chronic GVHD: From pathogenic B-cell receptor signaling to novel therapeutic targets. Blood. 2017;**129**(1):1-2

[6] Jagasia MH, Greinix HT, Arora M, Williams KM, Wolff D, Cowen EW, et al. National Institutes of Health Consensus Development Project on criteria for clinical trials in chronic graft-versus-host disease: I. The 2014 diagnosis and staging working group report. Journal of Biology of Blood Marrow Transplantation. 2015;**21**(3):389-401.e1

[7] Schoemans HM, Lee SJ, Ferrara JL, Wolff D, Levine JE, Schultz KR, et al. EBMT-NIH-CIBMTR task force position statement on standardized terminology & guidance for graft-versus-host disease assessment. Bone Marrow Transplantation. 2018;**53**(11):1401-1415

[8] Harris AC, Young R, Devine S, Hogan WJ, Ayuk F, Bunworasate U, et al. International, Multicenter Standardization of acute graft-versus-host disease clinical data collection: A report from the Mount Sinai acute GVHD international consortium. Biology of Blood and Marrow Transplantation. 2016;**22**(1):4-10

[9] D'Souza A, Fretham C, Lee SJ, Arora M, Brunner J, Chhabra S, et al. Current use of and trends in hematopoietic cell transplantation in the United States. Biology of Blood and Marrow Transplantation. 2020;**26**(8):e177-ee82

[10] Jamil MO, Mineishi S. State-of-the-art acute and chronic GVHD treatment. International Journal of Hematology. 2015;**101**(5):452-466

[11] Ramachandran V, Kolli SS, Strowd LC. Review of graft-versus-host disease. Dermatologic Clinics. 2019;**37**(4):569-582

[12] Jagasia M, Arora M, Flowers ME, Chao NJ, McCarthy PL, Cutler CS, et al. Risk factors for acute GVHD and survival after hematopoietic cell transplantation. Blood. 2012;**119**(1):296-307

[13] Zeiser R, Blazar BR. Acute graft-versus-host disease - Biologic process, prevention, and therapy. The New England Journal of Medicine. 2017;**377**(22):2167-2179

[14] Mathew NR, Vinnakota JM, Apostolova P, Erny D, Hamarsheh S, Andrieux G, et al. Graft-versus-host disease of the CNS is mediated by TNF upregulation in microglia. The Journal of Clinical Investigation. 2020;**130**(3):1315-1329

[15] Zeiser R, Teshima T. Nonclassical manifestations of acute GVHD. Blood. 2021;**138**(22):2165-2172

[16] Bhatt VR, Wang T, Chen K, Kitko CL, MacMillan ML, Pidala JA, et al. Chronic graft-versus-host disease, nonrelapse mortality, and disease relapse in older versus younger adults undergoing matched allogeneic peripheral blood hematopoietic cell transplantation: A Center for International Blood and Marrow Transplant Research Analysis. Transplantation and Cellular Therapy. 2022;**28**(1):34-42

[17] DeFilipp Z, Alousi AM, Pidala JA, Carpenter PA, Onstad LE, Arai S, et al. Nonrelapse mortality among patients diagnosed with chronic GVHD: An updated analysis from the Chronic GVHD Consortium. Blood Advances. 26 Oct 2021;**5**(20):4278-4284. DOI: 10.1182/bloodadvances.2021004941

[18] Bachier CR, Aggarwal SK, Hennegan K, Milgroom A, Francis K, Dehipawala S, et al. Epidemiology and treatment of chronic graft-versus-host disease post-allogeneic hematopoietic cell transplantation: A US claims analysis. Transplantation and Cellular Therapy. 2021;**27**(6):504.e1-504.e6

[19] Pavletic SZ, Martin PJ, Schultz KR, Lee SJ. The future of chronic graft-versus-host disease: Introduction to the 2020 National Institutes of Health Consensus Development Project Reports. Transplantation and Cellular Therapy. 2021;**27**(6):448-451

[20] Arai S, Arora M, Wang T, Spellman SR, He W, Couriel DR, et al. Increasing incidence of chronic graft-versus-host disease in allogeneic transplantation: A report from the Center for International Blood and Marrow Transplant Research. Biology of Blood and Marrow Transplantation. 2015;**21**(2):266-274

[21] Lee SJ. Classification systems for chronic graft-versus-host disease. Blood. 2017;**129**(1):30-37

[22] Zeiser R, Blazar BR. Pathophysiology of chronic graft-versus-host disease and therapeutic targets. The New England Journal of Medicine. 2017;**377**(26):2565-2579

[23] Hamilton BK. Updates in chronic graft-versus-host disease. Hematology American Society of Hematology Education Program. 2021;**2021**(1):648-654

[24] De Bosscher K, Vanden Berghe W, Beck IM, Van Molle W, Hennuyer N, Hapgood J, et al. A fully dissociated compound of plant origin for inflammatory gene repression. Proceedings of the National Academy of Sciences of the United States of America. 2005;**102**(44):15827-15832

[25] Wust S, Tischner D, John M, Tuckermann JP, Menzfeld C, Hanisch UK, et al. Therapeutic and adverse effects of a non-steroidal glucocorticoid receptor ligand in a mouse model of multiple sclerosis. PLoS One. 2009;**4**(12):e8202

[26] van Loo G, Sze M, Bougarne N, Praet J, Mc Guire C, Ullrich A, et al. Antiinflammatory properties of a plant-derived nonsteroidal, dissociated glucocorticoid receptor modulator in experimental autoimmune encephalomyelitis. Molecular Endocrinology (Baltimore, Md). 2010;**24**(2):310-322

[27] Gossye V, Elewaut D, Bougarne N, Bracke D, Van Calenbergh S, Haegeman G, et al. Differential mechanism of NF-kappaB inhibition by

two glucocorticoid receptor modulators in rheumatoid arthritis synovial fibroblasts. Arthritis and Rheumatism. 2009;**60**(11):3241-3250

[28] Rauner M, Thiele S, Sinningen K, Winzer M, Salbach-Hirsch J, Gloe I, et al. Effects of the selective glucocorticoid receptor modulator compound A on bone metabolism and inflammation in male mice with collagen-induced arthritis. Endocrinology. 2013;**154**(10):3719-3728

[29] Reuter KC, Grunwitz CR, Kaminski BM, Steinhilber D, Radeke HH, Stein J. Selective glucocorticoid receptor agonists for the treatment of inflammatory bowel disease: Studies in mice with acute trinitrobenzene sulfonic acid colitis. The Journal of Pharmacology and Experimental Therapeutics. 2012;**341**(1):68-80

[30] Reber LL, Daubeuf F, Plantinga M, De Cauwer L, Gerlo S, Waelput W, et al. A dissociated glucocorticoid receptor modulator reduces airway hyperresponsiveness and inflammation in a mouse model of asthma. Journal of Immunology. 2012;**188**(7):3478-3487

[31] Whitehouse MW. Anti-inflammatory glucocorticoid drugs: Reflections after 60 years. Inflammopharmacology. 2011;**19**(1):1-19

[32] Lesovaya E, Yemelyanov A, Swart AC, Swart P, Haegeman G, Budunova I. Discovery of compound A–A selective activator of the glucocorticoid receptor with anti-inflammatory and anti-cancer activity. Oncotarget. 2015;**6**(31):30730-30744

[33] Ruutu T, Gratwohl A, de Witte T, Afanasyev B, Apperley J, Bacigalupo A, et al. Prophylaxis and treatment of GVHD: EBMT-ELN working group recommendations for a standardized practice. Bone Marrow Transplantation. 2014;**49**(2):168-173

[34] Penack O, Marchetti M, Ruutu T, Aljurf M, Bacigalupo A, Bonifazi F, et al. Prophylaxis and management of graft versus host disease after stem-cell transplantation for haematological malignancies: Updated consensus recommendations of the European Society for Blood and Marrow Transplantation. The Lancet Haematology. 2020;**7**(2):e157-ee67

[35] Martin PJ, Rizzo JD, Wingard JR, Ballen K, Curtin PT, Cutler C, et al. First- and second-line systemic treatment of acute graft-versus-host disease: Recommendations of the American Society of Blood and Marrow Transplantation. Biology of Blood and Marrow Transplantation. 2012;**18**(8):1150-1163

[36] Mielcarek M, Furlong T, Storer BE, Green ML, McDonald GB, Carpenter PA, et al. Effectiveness and safety of lower dose prednisone for initial treatment of acute graft-versus-host disease: A randomized controlled trial. Haematologica. 2015;**100**(6):842-848

[37] Groth CG, Gahrton G, Lundgren G, Moller E, Pihlstedt P, Ringden O, et al. Successful treatment with prednisone and graft-versus-host disease in an allogeneic bone-marrow transplant recipient. Scandinavian Journal of Haematology. 1979;**22**(4):333-338

[38] Storb R, Kolb HJ, Graham TC, Kolb H, Weiden PL, Thomas ED. Treatment of established graft-versus-host disease in dogs by antithymocyte serum or prednisone. Blood. 1973;**42**(4):601-609

[39] Kendra J, Barrett AJ, Lucas C, Joshi R, Joss V, Desai M, et al. Response of graft versus host disease

to high doses of methyl prednisolone. Clinical and Laboratory Haematology. 1981;**3**(1):19-26

[40] Kanojia MD, Anagnostou AA, Zander AR, Vellekoop L, Spitzer G, Verma DS, et al. High-dose methylprednisolone treatment for acute graft-versus-host disease after bone marrow transplantation in adults. Transplantation. 1984;**37**(3):246-249

[41] Knop S, Hebart H, Gratwohl A, Kliem C, Faul C, Holler E, et al. Treatment of steroid-resistant acute GVHD with OKT3 and high-dose steroids results in better disease control and lower incidence of infectious complications when compared to high-dose steroids alone: A randomized multicenter trial by the EBMT chronic leukemia working party. Leukemia. 2007;**21**(8):1830-1833

[42] Quellmann S, Schwarzer G, Hubel K, Engert A, Bohlius J. Corticosteroids in the prevention of graft-vs-host disease after allogeneic myeloablative stem cell transplantation: A systematic review and meta-analysis. Leukemia. 2008;**22**(9):1801-1803

[43] Van Lint MT, Milone G, Leotta S, Uderzo C, Scime R, Dallorso S, et al. Treatment of acute graft-versus-host disease with prednisolone: Significant survival advantage for day +5 responders and no advantage for nonresponders receiving anti-thymocyte globulin. Blood. 2006;**107**(10):4177-4181

[44] Schacke H, Docke WD, Asadullah K. Mechanisms involved in the side effects of glucocorticoids. Pharmacology & Therapeutics. 2002;**96**(1):23-43

[45] Malard F, Huang XJ, Sim JPY. Treatment and unmet needs in steroid-refractory acute graft-versus-host disease. Leukemia. 2020;**34**(5):1229-1240

[46] Dignan FL, Clark A, Amrolia P, Cornish J, Jackson G, Mahendra P, et al. Diagnosis and management of acute graft-versus-host disease. British Journal of Haematology. 2012;**158**(1):30-45

[47] Inamoto Y, Martin PJ, Storer BE, Mielcarek M, Storb RF, Carpenter PA. Response endpoints and failure-free survival after initial treatment for acute graft-versus-host disease. Haematologica. 2014;**99**(2):385-391

[48] Xhaard A, Rocha V, Bueno B, de Latour RP, Lenglet J, Petropoulou A, et al. Steroid-refractory acute GVHD: Lack of long-term improved survival using new generation anticytokine treatment. Biology of Blood and Marrow Transplantation. 2012;**18**(3):406-413

[49] Martin PJ. How I treat steroid-refractory acute graft-versus-host disease. Blood. 2020;**135**(19):1630-1638

[50] Hill L, Alousi A, Kebriaei P, Mehta R, Rezvani K, Shpall E. New and emerging therapies for acute and chronic graft versus host disease. Therapeutic Advances in Hematology. 2018;**9**(1):21-46

[51] Martin PJ, Inamoto Y, Flowers ME, Carpenter PA. Secondary treatment of acute graft-versus-host disease: A critical review. Biology of Blood and Marrow Transplantation. 2012;**18**(7):982-988

[52] Zeiser R, von Bubnoff N, Butler J, Mohty M, Niederwieser D, Or R, et al. Ruxolitinib for glucocorticoid-refractory acute graft-versus-host disease. The New England Journal of Medicine. 2020;**382**(19):1800-1810

[53] Schroeder MA, Choi J, Staser K, DiPersio JF. The role of Janus kinase signaling in graft-versus-host disease and graft versus leukemia. Biology of Blood and Marrow Transplantation. 2018;**24**(6):1125-1134

[54] Jagasia M, Perales MA, Schroeder MA, Ali H, Shah NN, Chen YB, et al. Ruxolitinib for the treatment of steroid-refractory acute GVHD (REACH1): A multicenter, open-label phase 2 trial. Blood. 2020;**135**(20):1739-1749

[55] Zeiser R, Polverelli N, Ram R, Hashmi SK, Chakraverty R, Middeke JM, et al. Ruxolitinib for glucocorticoid-refractory chronic graft-versus-host disease. The New England Journal of Medicine. 2021;**385**(3):228-238

[56] Schroeder MA, Khoury HJ, Jagasia M, Ali H, Schiller GJ, Staser K, et al. A phase 1 trial of itacitinib, a selective JAK1 inhibitor, in patients with acute graft-versus-host disease. Blood Advances. 2020;**4**(8):1656-1669

[57] Zeiser R, Socié G, Schroeder MA, Abhyankar S, Vaz CP, Kwon M, et al. Efficacy and safety of itacitinib versus placebo in combination with corticosteroids for initial treatment of acute graft-versus-host disease (GRAVITAS-301): A randomised, multicentre, double-blind, phase 3 trial. The Lancet Haematology. 2022;**9**(1):e14-e25

[58] Groth C, van Groningen LFJ, Matos TR, Bremmers ME, Preijers F, Dolstra H, et al. Phase I/II trial of a combination of anti-CD3/CD7 immunotoxins for steroid-refractory acute graft-versus-host disease. Biology of Blood and Marrow Transplantation. 2019;**25**(4):712-719

[59] Socié G, Vigouroux S, Yakoub-Agha I, Bay JO, Fürst S, Bilger K, et al. A phase 3 randomized trial comparing inolimomab vs usual care in steroid-resistant acute GVHD. Blood. 2017;**129**(5):643-649

[60] Socié G, Milpied N, Yakoub-Agha I, Bay J-O, Fürst S, Bilger K, et al. Long-term follow-up of a phase 3 clinical trial of inolimomab for the treatment of primary steroid refractory aGVHD. Journal of Blood Advances. 2019;**3**(2):184-186

[61] Bouazzaoui A, Spacenko E, Mueller G, Miklos S, Huber E, Holler E, et al. Chemokine and chemokine receptor expression analysis in target organs of acute graft-versus-host disease. Genes and Immunity. 2009;**10**(8):687-701

[62] Couriel DR, Saliba R, de Lima M, Giralt S, Andersson B, Khouri I, et al. A phase III study of infliximab and corticosteroids for the initial treatment of acute graft-versus-host disease. Biology of Blood and Marrow Transplantation. 2009;**15**(12):1555-1562

[63] Nygaard M, Andersen NS, Moser CE, Olesen G, Schjødt IM, Heilmann C, et al. Evaluation of infliximab as second-line treatment of acute graft versus host disease -validating response on day 7 and 28 as predictors of survival. Bone Marrow Transplantation. 2018;**53**(7):844-851

[64] Busca A, Locatelli F, Marmont F, Ceretto C, Falda M. Recombinant human soluble tumor necrosis factor receptor fusion protein as treatment for steroid refractory graft-versus-host disease following allogeneic hematopoietic stem cell transplantation. American Journal of Hematology. 2007;**82**(1):45-52

[65] Khandelwal P, Emoto C, Fukuda T, Vinks AA, Neumeier L, Dandoy CE, et al. A prospective study of Alemtuzumab as a second-line agent for steroid-refractory acute graft-versus-host disease in pediatric and young adult allogeneic hematopoietic stem cell transplantation. Biology of Blood and Marrow Transplantation. 2016;**22**(12):2220-2225

[66] Bordigoni P, Dimicoli S, Clement L, Baumann C, Salmon A, Witz F, et al. Daclizumab, an efficient treatment for steroid-refractory acute graft-versus-host disease. British Journal of Haematology. 2006;**135**(3):382-385

[67] Soltani SN, Srinivasan R, Jerussi T, Barrett AJ, Hughes TE, Ramos C, et al. Long-term survival in patients with acute steroid refractory graft-versus-host-disease (SR-GVHD) treated with infliximab combined with daclizumab. Blood. 2013;**122**(21):4624

[68] Mo XD, Hong SD, Zhao YL, Jiang EL, Chen J, Xu Y, et al. Basiliximab for steroid-refractory acute graft-versus-host disease: A real-world analysis. American Journal of Hematology. 2022;**97**(4):458-469

[69] Coltoff A, Lancman G, Kim S, Steinberg A. Vedolizumab for treatment of steroid-refractory lower gastrointestinal acute graft-versus-host disease. Bone Marrow Transplantation. 2018;**53**(7):900-904

[70] Chen Y-B, Mohty M, Zeiser R, Teshima T, Jamy O, Maertens J, et al. Vedolizumab for the prevention of intestinal acute GVHD after allogeneic hematopoietic stem cell transplantation: A randomized phase 3 trial. Nature Medicine. 2024;**30**(8):2277-2287

[71] Mehta RS, Saliba RM, Jan A, Shigle TL, Wang E, Nieto Y, et al. Vedolizumab for steroid refractory lower gastrointestinal tract graft-versus-host disease. Transplantation and Cellular Therapy. 2021;**27**(3):272.e1-272.e5

[72] Bacigalupo A, Angelucci E, Raiola AM, Varaldo R, Di Grazia C, Gualandi F, et al. Treatment of steroid resistant acute graft versus host disease with an anti-CD26 monoclonal antibody—Begelomab. Bone Marrow Transplantation. 2020;**55**(8):1580-1587

[73] Bacigalupo A, Deeg HJ, Caballero D, Gualandi F, Raiola AM, Varaldo R, et al. Treatment of patients with steroid refractory acute graft vs host disease (SR-GvHD): A matched paired analysis of anti-CD26 (Begelomab) compared to other treatment. Blood. 2016;**128**(22):671

[74] Carpenter PA, Lowder J, Johnston L, Frangoul H, Khoury H, Parker P, et al. A phase II Multicenter study of visilizumab, humanized anti-CD3 antibody, to treat steroid-refractory acute graft-versus-host disease. Biology of Blood and Marrow Transplantation. 2005;**11**(6):465-471

[75] Carpenter PA, Appelbaum FR, Corey L, Deeg HJ, Doney K, Gooley T, et al. A humanized non–FcR-binding anti-CD3 antibody, visilizumab, for treatment of steroid-refractory acute graft-versus-host disease. Blood. 2002;**99**(8):2712-2719

[76] Antin JH, Ferrara JL. Cytokine dysregulation and acute graft-versus-host disease. Blood. 1992;**80**(12):2964-2968

[77] Marcondes AM, Hockenbery D, Lesnikova M, Dinarello CA, Woolfrey A, Gernsheimer T, et al. Response of steroid-refractory acute GVHD to α1-antitrypsin. Biology of Blood Marrow Transplantation. 2016;**22**(9):1596-1601

[78] Magenau JM, Goldstein SC, Peltier D, Soiffer RJ, Braun T, Pawarode A, et al. α1-antitrypsin infusion for treatment of steroid-resistant acute graft-versus-host disease. Blood, The Journal of the American Society of Hematology. 2018;**131**(12):1372-1379

[79] Benito AI, Furlong T, Martin PJ, Anasetti C, Appelbaum FR, Doney K, et al. Sirolimus (rapamycin) for the treatment of steroid-refractory acute graft-versus-host disease. Transplantation. 2001;**72**(12):1924-1929

[80] Biavasco F, Ihorst G, Wäsch R, Wehr C, Bertz H, Finke J, et al. Therapy response of glucocorticoid-refractory acute GVHD of the lower intestinal tract. Bone Marrow Transplantation. 2022;**57**(10):1500-1506

[81] Bolanos-Meade J, Jacobsohn DA, Margolis J, Ogden A, Wientjes MG, Byrd JC, et al. Pentostatin in steroid-refractory acute graft-versus-host disease. Journal of Clinical Oncology. 2005;**23**(12):2661-2668

[82] Holtan SG, Hoeschen A, Cao Q, Ustun C, Betts BC, Jurdi NE, et al. Phase II, open-label clinical trial of urinary-derived human chorionic gonadotropin/epidermal growth factor for life-threatening acute graft-versus-host disease. Transplantation and Cellular Therapy. 2023;**29**(8):509.e1-509.e8

[83] Holtan SG, Ustun C, Hoeschen A, Feola J, Cao Q, Gandhi P, et al. Phase 2 results of urinary-derived human chorionic gonadotropin/epidermal growth factor As treatment for life-threatening acute Gvhd. Blood. 2021;**138**(Suppl. 1):261

[84] Holtan SG, Hoeschen A, Cao Q, Arora M, Bachanova V, Brunstein CG, et al. Facilitating resolution of life-threatening acute graft-versus-host disease by supplementation of human chorionic gonadotropin and epidermal growth factor (Pregnyl): A phase I study. Blood. 2018;**132**(Suppl. 1):71

[85] Duvic M, Chiao N, Talpur R. Extracorporeal photopheresis for the treatment of cutaneous T-cell. Lymphoma. 2003;**7**(Suppl. 4):3-7

[86] Ali MM, Gedde-Dahl T, Osnes LT, Perrier F, Veierød MB, Tjønnfjord GE, et al. Extracorporeal photopheresis as graft-versus-host disease prophylaxis: A randomized controlled trial.

Transplantation and Cellular Therapy. 2023;**29**(6):364.e1-364e11

[87] Li D, Zhang J, Liu Z, Gong Y, Zheng Z. Human umbilical cord mesenchymal stem cell-derived exosomal miR-27b attenuates subretinal fibrosis via suppressing epithelial-mesenchymal transition by targeting HOXC6. Stem Cell Research & Therapy. 2021;**12**(1):24

[88] Thompson M, Mei SHJ, Wolfe D, Champagne J, Fergusson D, Stewart DJ, et al. Cell therapy with intravascular administration of mesenchymal stromal cells continues to appear safe: An updated systematic review and meta-analysis. EClinicalMedicine. 2020;**19**:100249

[89] Pidala J, Kitko C, Lee SJ, Carpenter P, Cuvelier GDE, Holtan S, et al. National Institutes of Health Consensus Development Project on Criteria for clinical trials in chronic graft-versus-host disease: IIb. The 2020 Preemptive therapy working group report. Transplantation and Cellular Therapy. 2021;**27**(8):632-641

[90] Ullah I, Subbarao RB, Rho GJ. Human mesenchymal stem cells - current trends and future prospective. Bioscience Reports. 28 Apr 2015;**35**(2):e00191. DOI: 10.1042/BSR20150025

[91] Galipeau J, Sensébé L. Mesenchymal stromal cells: Clinical challenges and therapeutic opportunities. Cell Stem Cell. 2018;**22**(6):824-833

[92] Rendra E, Scaccia E, Bieback K. Recent advances in understanding mesenchymal stromal cells. F1000Research. 27 Feb 2020;**9**:F1000 Faculty Rev-156. DOI: 10.12688/f1000research.21862.1

[93] Elgaz S, Kuçi Z, Kuçi S, Bönig H, Bader P. Clinical use of mesenchymal

stromal cells in the treatment of acute graft-versus-host disease. Transfusion Medicine and Hemotherapy : Offizielles Organ der Deutschen Gesellschaft fur Transfusionsmedizin und Immunhamatologie. 2019;**46**(1):27-34

[94] Voermans C, Hazenberg MD. Cellular therapies for graft-versus-host disease: A tale of tissue repair and tolerance. Blood, The Journal of the American Society of Hematology. 2020;**136**(4):410-417

[95] Godoy JAP, Paiva RMA, Souza AM, Kondo AT, Kutner JM, Okamoto OK. Clinical translation of mesenchymal stromal cell therapy for graft versus host disease. Frontiers in Cell and Developmental Biology. 2019;7:255

[96] Wu X, Jiang J, Gu Z, Zhang J, Chen Y, Liu X. Mesenchymal stromal cell therapies: Immunomodulatory properties and clinical progress. Stem Cell Research & Therapy. 2020;**11**(1):345

[97] Le Blanc K, Rasmusson I, Sundberg B, Götherström C, Hassan M, Uzunel M, et al. Treatment of severe acute graft-versus-host disease with third party haploidentical mesenchymal stem cells. The Lancet. 1 May 2004;**363**(9419):1439-1441. DOI: 10.1016/S0140-6736(04)16104-7

[98] Le Blanc K, Frassoni F, Ball L, Locatelli F, Roelofs H, Lewis I, et al. Mesenchymal stem cells for treatment of steroid-resistant, severe, acute graft-versus-host disease: A phase II study. The Lancet. 2008;**371**(9624):1579-1586

[99] Burnham AJ, Daley-Bauer LP, Horwitz EM. Mesenchymal stromal cells in hematopoietic cell transplantation. Blood Advances. 2020;**4**(22):5877-5887

[100] Zhao L, Chen S, Yang P, Cao H, Li L. The role of mesenchymal stem cells in hematopoietic stem cell transplantation: Prevention and treatment of graft-versus-host disease. Stem Cell Research & Therapy. 2019;**10**(1):182

[101] Murata M, Teshima T. Treatment of steroid-refractory acute graft-versus-host disease using commercial mesenchymal stem cell products. Frontiers in Immunology. 2021;**12**:724380

[102] Wright A, Arthaud-Day ML, Weiss ML. Therapeutic use of mesenchymal stromal cells: The need for inclusive characterization guidelines to accommodate all tissue sources and species. Frontiers in Cell and Developmental Biology. 2021;**9**:632717

[103] Mizukami A, Swiech K. Mesenchymal stromal cells: From discovery to manufacturing and commercialization. Stem Cells International. 2018;**2018**:4083921

[104] Kurtzberg J, Abdel-Azim H, Carpenter P, Chaudhury S, Horn B, Mahadeo K, et al. A phase 3, single-arm, prospective study of Remestemcel-L, ex vivo culture-expanded adult human mesenchymal stromal cells for the treatment of Pediatric patients who failed to respond to steroid treatment for acute graft-versus-host disease. Biology of Blood and Marrow Transplantation. 2020;**26**(5):845-854

[105] Trowsdale J, Betz AG. Mother's little helpers: Mechanisms of maternal-fetal tolerance. Nature Immunology. 2006;7(3):241-246

[106] Mori M, Bogdan A, Balassa T, Csabai T, Szekeres-Bartho J. The decidua-the maternal bed embracing the embryo-maintains the pregnancy. Seminars in Immunopathology. 2016;**38**(6):635-649

[107] Moll G, Ignatowicz L, Catar R, Luecht C, Sadeghi B, Hamad O, et al.

Different procoagulant activity of therapeutic mesenchymal stromal cells derived from bone marrow and placental decidua. Stem Cells Development. 2015;**24**(19):2269-2279

[108] Erkers T, Nava S, Yosef J, Ringdén O, Kaipe H. Decidual stromal cells promote regulatory T cells and suppress alloreactivity in a cell contact-dependent manner. Stem Cells and Development. 2013;**22**(19):2596-2605

[109] Karlsson H, Erkers T, Nava S, Ruhm S, Westgren M, Ringdén O. Stromal cells from term fetal membrane are highly suppressive in allogeneic settings in vitro. Clinical and Experimental Immunology. 2012;**167**(3):543-555

[110] Chang CJ, Yen ML, Chen YC, Chien CC, Huang HI, Bai CH, et al. Placenta-derived multipotent cells exhibit immunosuppressive properties that are enhanced in the presence of interferon-γ. Journal of Stem Cells. 2006;**24**(11):2466-2477

[111] Roelen DL, van der Mast BJ, In'tAnker PS, Kleijburg C, Eikmans M, van Beelen E, et al. Differential immunomodulatory effects of fetal versus maternal multipotent stromal cells. Human Immunology. 2009;**70**(1):16-23

[112] Croxatto D, Vacca P, Canegallo F, Conte R, Venturini PL, Moretta L, et al. Stromal cells from human decidua exert a strong inhibitory effect on NK cell function and dendritic cell differentiation. PLoS One. 2014;**9**(2):e89006

[113] Sadeghi B, Moretti G, Arnberg F, Samén E, Kohein B, Catar R, et al. Preclinical toxicity evaluation of clinical grade placenta-derived decidua stromal cells. Frontiers in Immunology. 2019;**10**:2685

[114] Sadeghi B, Witkamp M, Schefberger D, Arbman A, Ringdén O. Immunomodulation by placenta-derived decidua stromal cells. Role of histocompatibility, accessory cells and freeze–thawing. Cytotherapy. 2023;**25**(1):68-75

[115] Sadeghi B, Remberger M, Gustafsson B, Winiarski J, Moretti G, Khoein B, et al. Long-term follow-up of a pilot study using placenta-derived decidua stromal cells for severe acute graft-versus-host disease. Biology of Blood and Marrow Transplantation. 2019;**25**(10):1965-1969

[116] Ringdén O, Sadeghi B. Placenta-derived decidua stromal cells: A new frontier in the therapy of acute graft-versus-host disease. Stem Cells. 2024;**42**(4):291-300

[117] Alabdaljabar MS, Aslam HM, Veeraballi S, Faizee FA, Husain BH, Iqbal SM, et al. Restoration of the original inhabitants: A systematic review on fecal microbiota transplantation for graft-versus-host disease. Cureus. 6 Apr 2022;**14**(4):e23873. DOI: 10.7759/cureus.23873

[118] Qiao X, Biliński J, Wang L, Yang T, Luo R, Fu Y, et al. Safety and efficacy of fecal microbiota transplantation in the treatment of graft-versus-host disease. Bone Marrow Transplantation. 2023;**58**(1):10-19

[119] Rashidi A, Ebadi M, Rehman TU, Elhusseini H, Kazadi D, Halaweish H, et al. Potential of Fecal microbiota transplantation to prevent acute GVHD: Analysis from a phase II trial. Clinical Cancer Research. 2023;**29**(23):4920-4929

[120] Schub N, Günther A, Schrauder A, Claviez A, Ehlert C, Gramatzki M, et al. Therapy of steroid-refractory acute GVHD with CD52 antibody

alemtuzumab is effective. Bone Marrow
Transplantation. 2011;**46**(1):143-147

[121] Turner L. The American stem
cell sell in 2021: U.S. businesses
selling unlicensed and unproven stem
cell interventions. Cell Stem Cell.
2021;**28**(11):1891-1895

[122] Fendrick AM, Brixner D,
Rubin DT, Mease P, Liu H, Davis M,
et al. Sustained long-term benefits of
patient support program participation
in immune-mediated diseases: Improved
medication-taking behavior and lower
risk of a hospital visit. Journal of
Managed Care & Specialty Pharmacy.
2021;**27**(8):1086-1095

[123] Yalniz FF, Murad MH, Lee SJ,
Pavletic SZ, Khera N, Shah ND, et al.
Steroid refractory chronic graft-
versus-host disease: Cost-effectiveness
analysis. Biology of Blood and Marrow
Transplantation. 2018;**24**(9):1920-1927

[124] James A, Mannon RB. The cost
of transplant immunosuppressant
therapy: Is this sustainable?
Current Transplantation Reports.
2015;**2**(2):113-121

[125] Bachier CR, Skaar JR, Dehipawala S,
Miao B, Ieyoub J, Taitel H. Budget impact
analysis of belumosudil for chronic
graft-versus-host disease treatment in
the United States. Journal of Medical
Economics. 2022;**25**(1):857-863

[126] Holtan SG, Hoeschen AL, Cao Q,
Arora M, Bachanova V, Brunstein CG,
et al. Facilitating resolution of life-
threatening acute GVHD with human
chorionic gonadotropin and epidermal
growth factor. Blood Advances.
2020;**4**(7):1284-1295

Chapter 5

Application of Mesenchymal Stem Cells in Graft-Versus-Host Disease as a Regenerative Therapy

Neslihan Mandacı Şanlı and Aysu Timuroğlu

Abstract

Graft versus host disease (GVHD) is a complication that significantly affects mortality and morbidity after hematopoietic stem cell transplantation (HSCT), and corticosteroids are the most commonly used first-line treatment for GVHD worldwide. However, approximately half of GVHD cases develop non-responsiveness to corticosteroid therapy, and despite new developments in the field of GVHD, it is not clear which treatment agent will be used as the first choice in the second-line setting. Mesenchymal stem cells (MSCs) are multipotent progenitor cells that can be derived from many tissues such as bone marrow, fetal structures, and muscle are self-renewing and have the capacity to differentiate into many different tissues. The administration of MSCs in the treatment of immune system-related diseases has recently become popular due to their immune suppressive and immune-modulatory properties, and clinical studies on MSCs have been focused. Since GVHD is also an immune-related tissue damage and systemic inflammation, the use of MSC infusion in the treatment of GVHD has attracted the attention of clinicians. Many trials have been published on this subject. In this review, we analyzed the publications on the application of MSCs in patients with GVHD and investigated the efficacy of MSCs in the treatment of GVHD.

Keywords: graft versus host disease, mesenchymal stem cells, hematopoietic stem cell transplantation, immune modulation, immune suppression

1. Introduction

1.1 Mesenchymal stem cells

"Mesenchymal stem cells" (MSCs) are adult non-hematopoietic stem cells and are multipotent, self-renewing, heterogeneous cells with fibroblast-like morphology and multilineage differentiation capacity [1, 2]. Mesenchymal stem cells (MSCs) were first identified by Alexander Friedenstein in the late 1960s, and their pharmacological application in humans was first investigated in 1995 [3, 4]. They can be isolated from many tissues such as bone marrow, adipose tissue, muscle, peripheral blood, hair follicles, teeth, placenta and umbilical cord, Wharton's gel, amniotic fluid, amniotic membranes, dental pulp, synovial fluid [5–7]. Although mesenchymal stem cells (MSCs) exhibit distinct characteristics based on the tissue of origin, they are required to fulfill the three minimum criteria established by the "International Society for Cellular Therapy" (ISCT) in 2006. The first criterion stipulates that MSCs must adhere to plastic surfaces when cultured *in vitro*. Secondly, MSCs must express surface antigens CD73, CD90, and CD105 while lacking the expression of "CD45, CD34, CD14 or CD11b, CD79a or CD19, and HLA-DR". The final criterion mandates that mesenchymal stem cells (MSCs) must exhibit the capacity to differentiate into mesodermal lineages, such as adipocytes, chondrocytes, and osteoblasts, under *in vitro* culture conditions [8]. Additionally, MSCs can be efficiently obtained from peripheral blood and adipose tissue through minimally invasive methods [1, 9]. Some ethical issues may restrict the use of MSCs for therapeutic purposes. The collection of bone marrow-derived or adipose tissue-derived stem cells is easier than umbilical cord-derived stem cells, which are collected autologously from the patient [10].

First of all, the process of collection of MSCs may cause pain in the donor, impairment of donor comfort, and donor morbidity. In addition, during *in vitro* processing of the MSCs, the capacity for differentiation may be reduced.

Furthermore, the differentiation potential of mesenchymal stem cells (MSCs) may be influenced by various environmental factors, including age, stress, and genetic variations [3]. Because of all these problems, obtaining MSCs from embryonic tissues such as umbilical cord and umbilical cord blood, fetal tissues, and placenta is preferred over other sources of MSCs and causes less ethical problems [11–14]. In clinical trials, bone marrow, cord blood, peripheral blood, and adipose tissue are used for obtaining MSCs, and apheresis procedure is applied after G-CSF induction if MSCs are to be obtained from peripheral blood. If MSCs are to be obtained from bone marrow and cord blood, they are collected directly from the source. After these cells are collected from their source, they are isolated, cultured, and proliferated in special media [15]. In many clinical trials, the average dose of MSC infusion in humans is 1–2 million hc/kg and does not exceed 12 million hc/kg. The doses of MSCs vary between species, and factors such as preparation and dosing of the MSCs may alter their paracrine effects. In particular, the infusions of MSCs derived from bone marrow and adipose tissue are the safest ones, and side effects such as febrile reactions are the least common [4]. Mesenchymal stem cells (MSCs) possess the ability to differentiate not only into mesodermal cell lineages but also into a variety of other tissue types. They have the capacity to differentiate not only into cells originating from the mesoderm leaflet but also into other cell types originating from both the ectoderm and endodermal leaflet (e.g., neurons, cardiomyocytes, and hepatocytes) [16–19]. This is called plasticity and is utilized in cell regeneration [1]. Although mesenchymal stem cells have a similar phenotype, they have a heterogeneous biological structure and function. Their different growth and differentiation capacities and pro-angiogenic properties cause this heterogeneity. For example, when an adipose tissue- or bone marrow-derived MSC is compared with a fetal-derived MSC, it has been found that MSCs isolated from fetal tissues have higher proliferation capacity, longer survival, greater differentiation capacity, and lower immunogenicity [3, 10]. Umbilical cord-derived MSCs are richer in angiogenic factors, which makes them preferable to bone marrow-derived MSCs [10]. This may be an important factor in the different results of clinical trials.

Mesenchymal stem cells have recently been a popular subject of research with the application of therapeutic cellular products in the clinic. Features such as migration to damaged tissues, immunotrophic functions, and tissue regeneration/repair have led to the inclusion of MSCs among the treatment options in the treatment of immunologic/inflammatory diseases and extensive studies on this subject have been carried out [3]. In addition, they have the ability to induce angiogenesis, promote cell survival, and inhibit the immune system [20]. The bioactive agents massively secreted from MSCs have both immune-modulatory and trophic properties and are used clinically in patients with rejection after HSCT due to their immunosuppressive properties [1, 2].

All of these advantages of MSCs have brought their use in regenerative medicine and in the treatment of many diseases to the agenda. In this article, we tried to present a review of the use of MSCs in GVHD and contribute to the literature.

1.2 Graft versus host disease

"Hematopoietic stem cell transplantation" (HSCT) is a high-intensity therapeutic approach employed in the treatment of both malignant and non-malignant hematologic disorders, immune system diseases, certain solid tumors, and metabolic conditions. This procedure aims to restore the hematopoietic and immune functions of hematopoietic progenitor cells. To date, approximately 1.5 million HSCT procedures have been conducted globally [21]. Thanks to innovations in transplant regimens and better supportive care, survival rates of patients with HSCT have increased. The most important complication limiting the use of allogeneic HSCT in the treatment of hematologic malignancies is graft versus host disease (GVHD). It is one of the most important barriers affecting the success of hematopoietic stem cell transplantation and is the most important cause of mortality and morbidity after transplantation. Disease relapse, graft rejection, and acute or chronic GVHD are the most common complications after HSCT [22, 23].

Graft versus host disease is a systemic inflammatory response caused by donor T cells recognizing foreign cells of the recipient and immune dysregulation after HSCT, which occurs when autoreactive immune cells trigger inflammation. Donor lymphocytes perceive the recipient as foreign, which causes systemic inflammation. Activated T cells attempt to destroy antigen-bearing cells in the recipient, which can result in an immunologic response that can cause severe organ damage [21]. GVHD presents as two different clinical conditions, acute and chronic. It is classified as acute/chronic GVHD according to its clinical presentation and its development in the first 100 days and beyond after allogeneic HSCT [24]. In 2005, acute and chronic GVHD was defined according to clinical findings in the National Institutes of Health Consensus Criteria Development Project [25, 26]. According to NIH criteria, GVHD is divided into four subgroups: (1) classic acute graft versus host disease (GVHD) is characterized by the absence of diagnostic and distinctive features of chronic GVHD (cGVHD), with clinical manifestations occurring within 100 days following allogeneic hematopoietic stem cell transplantation (allo-HSCT) or donor lymphocyte infusion (DLI). (2) Persistent and/or recurrent late-onset acute GVHD presents with the clinical characteristics of classic acute GVHD but without the diagnostic features of cGVHD, appearing beyond 100 days after allo-HSCT or DLI. (3) Classic cGVHD can develop at any time following HSCT and is defined by the presence of diagnostic and distinctive characteristics of cGVHD without concurrent acute GVHD. (4) Overlap syndrome, on the other hand, is distinguished by the simultaneous presence of clinical features associated with both acute GVHD and cGVHD [27, 28]. The diagnosis of chronic graft versus host disease (cGVHD) requires the presence of at least one diagnostic manifestation or at least one distinctive manifestation confirmed through biopsy, laboratory testing, or radiographic evaluation in the same or a different tissue [22]. Currently, 30–50% of allogeneic bone marrow transplant recipients have acute

GVHD, and 30–70% have CR GVHD. Despite calcineurin inhibitors and methotrexate prophylaxis, GVHD is still common and corticosteroids are used as first-line treatment [29]. However, new treatment approaches need to be developed due to increasing steroid resistance [21]. Mortality rates are higher in steroid-refractory patients, and many agents such as mycophenolate mofetil, JAK inhibitors, extracorporeal photopheresis, sirolimus, and everolimus have been introduced in second-line treatment. Despite all these options, an optimal option in corticosteroid unresponsive/refractory cases has still not been developed [24, 30]. Recently published and investigated therapies for GVHD target inflammatory pathways and the most important disadvantage of these therapies is that they also increase immunodeficiency. Many studies have been published on the use of MSCs in the treatment of both acute and chronic GVHD due to their immune system-related effects.

2. MSCs and immune modulation

The tissue repair and immune suppressive effects of "mesenchymal stem cells" have brought their use in the treatment of GVHD to the agenda. These cells, which have immune modulatory, low immunogenicity, and homing properties, are promising in the treatment of immune-related diseases and inflammatory diseases [31]. By preventing the development of an exaggerated immune response, MSCs exert a general immunosuppressive effect [32]. Immune dysfunction such as inadequate or exaggerated immune response plays a role in the pathogenesis of many diseases. MSCs also show immunomodulatory effects by direct cell contact with immune system cells or by the release of cytokines, growth factors, etc. as a result of paracrine effects and seem to be effective in the treatment of diseases with immune dysfunction in their pathogenesis [32].

MSCs have attracted an interest for their therapeutic capabilities beyond GVHD treatment, which includes use in cancer treatment and regenerative medicine. Hmadcha et al. underscored the role of MSCs in cancer therapy and immune regulation due to their anti-inflammatory and immunomodulatory properties that may be mediated by the secretion of bioactive molecules [1]. Furthermore, MSCs can change the tumor microenvironment, inhibit tumor development, and increase anti-tumor response, which is important for HSCT treatment of most hematologic cancers [1]. At the same time, MSC-based therapies are investigated for treatment of autoimmune and neurodegenerative conditions which demonstrates versatile immune modulatory properties [3].

MSCs can affect both innate and adaptive immune system cells. By decreasing the release of IL-2/IL-15, IFN-γ, MSCs inhibit the proliferation, differentiation, and activation of natural killer (NK) cells involved in the innate immune response and CD4 and CD8 positive T cells involved in the adaptive immune response, leading to immune suppression. Adhesion molecules such as ICAM-1 and VCAM-1 are highly expressed on the surface of MSCs, and these adhesion molecules play a role in the interaction of MSCs and T-reg cells. T-reg cells are primitive T cells with anti-inflammatory and immunomodulatory properties, and MSCs cause immune tolerance by increasing the number of T-reg cells [33–37]. Moreover, various studies indicate that MSCs modulated the immune response by interacting directly with immune cells and by releasing immunoregulatory molecules in extracellular vesicles (EVs) [38]. Mendiratta et al. reported that MSC-derived EVs with microRNAs and cytokines can alter the inflammatory response of the host and increase immune tolerance, thereby controlling the GVHD [2]. These results broaden the scope for MSC-based therapies where EVs may serve as a cell-free substitute for MSCs and reduce the risks with live cell transplantation without sacrificing the therapeutic effect [2].

In vivo studies have demonstrated that human-derived MSCs inhibit allogeneic T-cell proliferation. Activation and differentiation of Th17 and Th1, which are pro-inflammatory cells, are inhibited by PGE2 released from the MSCs [32]. As a result, more than 30 cytokines such as TGF-β, hepatocyte growth factor (HGF), PGE2, IL-6, and NO. are secreted by MSCs and are involved in T cell immune modulation [38]. At the same time, they can suppress the proliferation, maturation, and antibody production of B cells. In a study conducted by Glennie et al., it was shown that B cell proliferation was paused in the G0/G1 phase when B cells and MSCs were co-cultured. In addition, IL-1RA and CCL2 released from MSCs can block B cell maturation and immunoglobulin production. In addition, MSC treatment is important in tissue reconstruction owing to its potency in stimulating angiogenesis while reducing fibrosis. According to the report by Merimi et al., MSC secretes both vascular endothelial growth factor (VEGF) and hepatocyte growth factor (HGF), which aid endothelial cells to survive and regenerate, thus serving an important function of organ protection in GVHD patients [3]. These features of MSCs, in addition to the antiviral effects, enable the use of mesenchymal cells in treatment of HSCT-associated problems like GVHD [3]. If we look at the effect of MSCs on macrophages, by suppressing the release of pro-inflammatory cytokines such as TNF-α and IL-1 β, increasing COX2 and prostaglandin E2 synthesis and causing IL-10 production in macrophages, they reduce the phagocytosis of macrophages and produce an anti-inflammatory effect [39]. MSCs also have special functions known as sensors and switchers of the immune system, triggering inflammation by activating the immune system when it is inhibited and stopping inflammation when the immune system is over-activated. There is a balance between MSCs and the immune system regulating tissue homeostasis and inflammatory response [10].

Moreover, MSCs have been reported to show the ability to differentiate into many other types of cells, which adds to their potential therapeutic value. Research demonstrated the possibility of MSCs differentiating into hepatocyte, neuronal, and epithelial cells, which aids in the repair of tissues in organs damaged due to GVHD like liver, gut, and skin [16–18]. He and Nagamura-Inoue have pointed out the beneficial factors of umbilical cord MSCs, which are more immunostimulatory and less immunogenic as compared to bone marrow MSCs, thereby making them a good source for allogenic transplants [7]. These studies are in line with the idea of employing various sources of MSCs to improve the treatment effectiveness and reduce the chances of immune rejection [7].

The fact that MSCs have both immune-suppressive and immune-modulatory properties has brought to the agenda the investigation of the effects of MSCs use in GVHD cases occurring after HSCT, which is an immune event. In recent studies, it is noteworthy that MSCs may reduce the severity of chronic GVHD and the incidence of acute GVHD after HSCT [21]. Here, we aimed to have an idea about the efficacy of MSC therapy in GVHD patients by reviewing the studies on the use of MSCs in individuals with GVHD.

3. Evidence of MSCs application in GVHD

"Hematopoietic stem cell transplantation" has emerged as the preferred treatment for hematologic malignancies and genetic disorders, driven by the growing utilization of haploidentical bone marrow transplants and advancements in transplant-related outcomes. "According to the Center for International Blood and Marrow Transplant Research", over 60,000 hematopoietic stem cell transplantations (HSCTs) are performed annually. Graft versus host disease (GVHD) remains the most critical and potentially fatal complication of HSCT, persisting as a significant challenge despite advancements in transplantation technologies, the development of new therapeutic agents, and improved prophylactic strategies [40, 41]. A wide variety of therapeutic strategies are being developed to prevent and treat the development of GVHD. "Anti-thymocyte globülin" (ATG) and "anti-lymphocyte globülin" (ALG), antibodies against T cells, have been used *in vivo* to prevent the development of GVHD. However, while neither treatment has a positive contribution to survival, they are effective in reducing the frequency of GVHD. Corticosteroids are the gold standard in GVHD treatment due to their anti-lymphocyte and anti-inflammatory effects [42]. However, half of GVHD patients under steroid treatment go into complete remission while the rest are steroid-refractory and have poor survival [23]. Despite many advances in the field of HSCT, there is still not enough progress in the field of GVHD to reduce mortality and morbidity. In patients with severe GVHD, survival rates are 25% in grade 3 and only 5% in grade 4 patients [43, 44]. Allogeneic transplantation is an increasingly practiced and preferred treatment modality, and new approaches to reduce the development of GVHD are needed. "Mesenchymal stem cell therapy", a cell-based therapy, is one of the promising approaches in the treatment of GVHD due to its immunomodulatory effects [45, 46]. MSCs can cause genetic modification by causing overexpression/blockage of specific genes and act as immune modulators by increasing/decreasing the immune response [32].

Mesenchymal stem cells are able to migrate to the damaged area and help tissue repair by releasing bioactive substances with antapoptotic, angiogenic, anti-inflammatory, anti-fibrotic, immunomodulatory, and anti-oxidant effects. Since these properties have been known, MSCs have become target molecules in the treatment of regenerative medicine and immune diseases, for example, the use of MSCs in the treatment of many diseases such as Crohn's disease, GVHD, neurodegenerative diseases, aplastic anemia, etc. is on the agenda [2]. The fact that MSCs can down-express MHC Class 1 molecules and do not contain MHC Class II molecules allows them to form a barrier to immune rejection, facilitates their application even without donor-recipient HLA compatibility, and increases their immunoregulatory effects through cell–cell contact [47–50]. Mesenchymal stem cells have two important properties: maintaining tissue homeostasis and enabling engraftment. Depending on the extent of inflammation and their stimulation by toll-like receptors, MSCs may have pro-inflammatory and anti-inflammatory properties [51]. In GVHD cases, they cause immune suppression through a reaction called efferocytosis. MSCs lead to activation of cytotoxic T lymphocytes and natural killer (NK) cells, which results in apoptosis, followed by clearance of dead MSCs by monocytes and dendritic cells, called efferocytosis [52–54]. This results in the release of immune suppressive mediators "HLA-G, prostaglandin E2 (PgE2), indoleamine-2-3-dioxygenase (IDO), transforming growth factor-beta (TGF-β), cyclooxygenase 2 (COX-2), programmed cell death-ligand 1 (PD-L1), interleukin (IL)-1RA, IL-10, IL-6, CCL2". Apoptosis and efferocytosis are essential for the immune modulation induced by MSCs in patients with GVHD [2]. With the realization of the immune modulatory potential of MSCs, their use in the treatment of immune system-related diseases in the clinic has come to the fore and clinical studies have started to be conducted in this field. Especially studies on their use in the prevention and treatment of GVHD have been focused.

For the first time, Bartholomew showed that the survival of skin grafts increased with the use of mesenchymal stem cells [55]. Since then, many studies have been conducted on mesenchymal stem cells, and it has been shown that they inhibit the proliferation and function of T cells, B cells, dendritic cells, and natural killer cells, and their immunomodulatory effects have been confirmed [23]. Studies have also published that mesenchymal stem cells are part of the niche, support hematopoiesis, and thus have an active role in facilitating the engraftment of hematopoietic stem cells after transplantation [56, 57]. However, the results of studies on the clinical use of MSCs in cases with GVHD are contradictory [23]. When we look at the literature, we come across a large number of publications on the use of MSCs in acute GVHD cases, while data on the use of MSCs in patients with chronic GVHD are limited. The reason for this can be interpreted as that the responses to MSC therapy in acute GVHD are better than in chronic GVHD [58]. In a retrospective review, we see that there is experience with the use of MSC in about 1400 patients with acute GVHD [2]. Firstly, in 2004, Le Blanc et al. at the Karolinska Institute in Sweden published that a 9-year-old male child with steroid-refractory severe acute GVHD (grade IV) had a complete response after MSC infusion, and then many studies were conducted one after another to investigate the possible benefits of MSCs [2, 23]. Currently, there are 62 studies reported in the clinical trials related to MSCs and GVHD (the list of the completed trials is shown in **Table 1**).

In this first case reported in the literature, the patient received allogeneic (from the mother) bone marrow-derived MSCs as two serial infusions, and a complete response (CR) was not achieved in the first infusion. CR was achieved after the second infusion, and the patient lived a healthy life for 1 year [47, 59]. In another 32-patient study conducted by Kebriae et al., bone marrow-derived MSCs were administered as two serial infusions to patients with acute GVHD grade II-IV, and corticosteroids were given concomitantly. In this study, 77% of patients had a complete response and 16% had a partial response, and none of these patients had an infusion-related reaction [60]. If we look at the stem cell source in the stem cell studies performed with acute GVHD, not only bone marrow-derived MSCs were used, but Wharton gel was used as a source of MSCs in Soder et al.'s study of 10 patients who developed acute GVHD after allogeneic HSCT in 2020. The "overall response rate" (ORR) was 70%, with CR in four patients and PR in three patients [61].

In 2021, Murata et al. administered a commercial molecule called "Ryoncil™" (remestemcel-L), a bone marrow-derived MSC product, in patients with steroid-resistant acute GVHD, but no superiority to placebo was achieved. Nevertheless, it was approved for use in pediatric patients in New Zealand and Canada based on the results of a subgroup analysis (OR rates were significantly higher in a small group of pediatric patients with liver infiltration). The remestemcel-L equivalent, Temcell®, was first used in Japan in 2016 for the treatment of regenerative diseases and was effective in 381 patients [30].

In 2019, Zhao et al. examined 10 multicenter studies published between 2008 and 2017 on the use of MSCs in patients with acute GVHD. All patients who participated in these studies underwent HSCT for malignant hematologic disease, and some of the patients received MSC infusion, while others did not receive it. The patients received a single infusion of MSCs to prevent the development of GVHD, whereas multiple infusions were given for therapeutic purposes. The MSC infusion was administered before/after HSCT. With this meta-analysis, it was concluded that MSC infusion may reduce the incidence of chronic GVHD and is effective in prolonging CR rates and survival in patients with acute GVHD [23].

Trial	Study title	Source	Phase	Patients	Completion	Country
NCT01956903	"Treatment of Refractory Acute Graft-Versus-Host Disease by Sequential Infusion of Allogenic Mesenchymal Stem Cell. (CSM/EICH2010)"	"Allogenic mesenchymal stem cells"	1–2	18–65	2013–2109	Spain
NCT02824653	"Allogenic Bone Marrow Mesenchymal Stem Cells Infusion in Patients With Steroid-refractory GVHD"	"BM-derived"	1–2	1–65 years	2016–2112	Pakistan
NCT01222039	"Multicenter Clinical Trial for the Evaluation of Mesenchymal Stem Cells From Adipose Tissue in Patients With Chronic Graft Versus Host Disease. (CMM/EICH/2008"	"Allogenic mesenchymal stem cells"	1–2	18–65 years	2014–2106	Spain
NCT02687646	"MSC for Graft Versus Host Disease Treatment"	"Adipose tissue derived"	1–2	18–65 years	2022–2101	Spain
NCT00284986	"Safety and Efficacy of Prochymal® for the Salvage of Treatment-Refractory Acute GVHD Patients"	"Prochymal® (Ex-vivo Cultured Adult Human Mesenchymal Stem Cells)"	2	6 months–70 years	2007–2102	United States
NCT00827398	"Treatment of Steroid Resistant GVHD by Infusion MSC (MSCforGVHD)"	"Mesenchymal Stem Cells Expanded With Human Plasma and Platelet Lysate"	1–2	1–68 years	2013–2107	Netherlands
NCT00366145	"Efficacy and Safety of Adult Human Mesenchymal Stem Cells to Treat Steroid Refractory Acute Graft Versus Host Disease (GVHD)"	"Prochymal®"	3	6 month–70 years	2009–5	United States
NCT00504803	"Mesenchymal Stem Cell Infusion as Prevention for Graft Rejection and Graft-versus-host Disease"	"PBSC or cord blood"	2	Up to 75 years	2010–2012	Belgium
NCT02923375	"A Study of CYP-001 for the Treatment of Steroid-Resistant Acute Graft Versus Host Disease"	"Mesenchymoangioblast-derived mesenchymal stem cells"	1	18–70 years	2020–2106	Australia
NCT00136903	"Safety and Efficacy Study of Adult Human Mesenchymal Stem Cells to Treat Acute Graft Versus Host Disease (GVHD)"	"Ex-vivo cultured adult human mesenchymal stem cells (hMSCs) (Prochymal®)"	2	18–70 years	2008–2107	United States
NCT01318330	"Safety Study of Homeo-GH (Bone Marrow Derived Clonal Mesenchymal Stem Cell) to Treat Acute/Chronic Graft Versus Host Disease (GVHD) (Homeo-GH)"	"Bone marrow derivated"	1	≥18 years	2012–2106	Republic of Korea

Trial	Study title	Source	Phase	Patients	Completion	Country
NCT04738981	"Efficacy and Safety of UC-MSCs for the Treatment of Steroid-resistant aGVHD Following Allo-HSCT"	"Umbilical cord-derived"	3	18–70 years	2023–2105	China
NCT00562497	"Efficacy and Safety of Prochymal® Infusion in Combination With Corticosteroids for the Treatment of Newly Diagnosed Acute Graft Versus Host Disease (GVHD)"	"Prochymal®"	3	18–70 years	2010–5	United States
NCT03106662	"Mesenchymal Stem Cell Infusion in Haploidentical Hematopoietic Stem Cell Transplantation in Patients With Hematological Malignancies"	"Bone marrow derivated"	3	≥18 years	2017–2110	Turkey
NCT00361049	"Donor Mesenchymal Stem Cell Infusion in Treating Patients With Acute or Chronic Graft-Versus-Host Disease After Undergoing a Donor Stem Cell Transplant"		1	≥18 years	2010–2011	United States
NCT00823316	"Safety and Efficacy Study of Umbilical Cord Blood-Drived Mesenchymal Stem Cells to Promote Engraftment of Unrelated Hematopoietic Stem Cell Transplantation"	"Umblical cord derivated"	1–2	2–19 years	2010–2102	Republic of Korea
NCT06469411	"Effect of PMSCs and Their Secretome for the Treatment of GvHD (GvHD)"	"Placenta"	3	16–50 years	2024–2101	Islamic Republic of Iran
NCT02336230	"A Prospective Study of Remestemcel-L, Ex-vivo Cultured Adult Human Mesenchymal Stromal Cells, for the Treatment of Pediatric Participants Who Have Failed to Respond to Steroid Treatment for Acute Graft-Versus-Host Disease (aGVHD)"	"Remestemcel-L"	3	2 months-17 years	2018–2104	United States

Table 1.
The completed trials about mesenchymal stem cells and graft versus host disease at ClinicalTrials.gov

Recent research has dealt with the importance of mitochondria transfer between MSCs and damaged immune cells in the context of GVHD patients. Li et al. showed that MSCs are capable of transferring mitochondria to the immune cells of the host through gap junctions, which aids in the restoration of immune balance and more effective tissue repair [50]. This may give part of the explanation for the therapeutic effect of MSCs in GVHD treatment. Also, MSC apoptosis, followed by efferocytosis from the recipient's immune cells, has been suggested to be an important immuno-suppressive mechanism in GVHD. Galleu et al. demonstrated that apoptotic MSCs stimulate the production of PGE2, altering the immune response to one of tolerance, which decreases inflammation in the GVHD patient [52].

In another study conducted by Shafeghat et al. in 2023, it was shown that GVHD-related symptoms and signs decreased and survival increased in patients who developed GVHD after HSCT by administering exosomes derived from the MSCs, but not the MSCs themselves, to patients with GVHD. Exosomes are 30–120 nm in diameter and carry biologically active molecules. These molecules play a key role in the immunosuppressive and paracrine effects of MSCs in tissue repair and therapeutic efficacy and can easily pass through physiologic barriers thanks to their easy preparation procedures and small, liquid structure. They are safer molecules than stem cell-based therapies. In patients with GVHD, it has been demonstrated that the use of exosomes originating from MSCs inhibits IFN-γ and TNF-α release with NK cell activation and reduces the lethal properties of NK cells and inflammatory responses [22].

In a phase II/III clinical trial conducted by Muroi et al., bone marrow-derived MSC administration improved the survival of patients without side effects [62]. Similarly, in a phase II clinical study published by Frederic Baron et al. in 2010, a cohort population of 20 patients with hematologic malignancies was infused with three doses of MSCs. Graft rejection developed in 1 patient, but permanent engraftment was achieved in the remaining 19 patients. In total, 35% of patients developed acute GVHD grade II-IV, while 65% developed moderate/severe chronic GVHD. At the end of 1 year, the "overall survival" (OS) was 80% and progression-free survival (PFS) was 60%, demonstrating a reduction in GVHD mortality without a reduction in graft versus tumor effect in patients with hematologic malignancies [63].

The actions of MSCs have also been corroborated by Cheung et al., who identified particular biomarkers of MSC activity in patients with GVHD and their correspond-ing clinical outcomes. It was shown that the levels of PGE2 and IL-10 after infusion of MSCs are associated with clinical outcomes achieved after MSC infusion and thus confirmed the immunomodulatory abilities of MSCs in GVHD management [53, 54]. Moreover, Bernardo and Fibbe pointed out that MSCs are able to alter their immu-nosuppressive functions in accordance with the level of inflammation as they are "sensors and switchers" of the inflammatory process [51]. This makes MSC therapy complex and highly individualistic with the possibilities of specific patient factors determining the outcome of the treatment.

In 2016, in a recently published meta-analysis, positive results were obtained with the use of MSCs, and it was shown that there was a 6-month survival advantage with MSC treatment in aGVHD cases. However, controlled studies supporting these results have not been published, and there is inconsistency between the results of studies on the benefit of MSCs in GVHD prevention [59, 64–66]. More studies are needed to determine whether there is a clinical benefit of MSCs in the treatment and prevention of GVHD. The number of studies on the use of MSCs in patients with chronic GVHD is limited and overall response rates have been found in a wide range. The number of patients in these studies is quite small, and studies with larger populations are needed to obtain more reliable results [53].

In view of the optimistic yet inconsistent results of MSC treatment, MSC source selection optimization and dosing regimens alongside existing immunosuppressive therapies offer immense possibilities for future research. The further development of MSC exosomes and MSCs provides an opportunity to increase the therapeutic efficacy of GVHD while alleviating side effects [55, 56]. Moreover, biomarker standardization will enable better patient stratification and treatment customization in GVHD patients where MSCs are infused, thereby achieving more reliable responses [53]. In allogeneic HSCT, co-transplantation of MSCs with the graft may promote engraftment, improve OS and CR, and reduce the risk of chronic GVHD. However, it is less effective in reducing the risk of developing acute GVHD and non-relapse mortality. In patients with chronic GVHD, IL-10 secreted from MSCs induces cd5-positive regulatory B cell formation and provides immune suppression by reducing inflammatory cytokine-producing T cell production [2, 67, 68].

In a meta-analysis conducted by Morata et al. on the use of MSCs in prophylaxis of chronic GVHD, it was shown that prophylactic use of bone marrow/umbilical cord-derived MSCs in pediatric and adult age group HSCT recipients may decrease the incidence of chronic GVHD and increase survival [69]. In 2010, Weng et al. conducted the first study on the use of bone marrow-derived MSCs in patients with refractory chronic GVHD after allogeneic HSCT. In the study, 14 of 19 patients (73.5% responded), 10 of them had CR and 4 patients had PR response. No side effects were observed in any of the patients during or after MSC infusion. In this study, 2-year survival was 77.7% and the idea that the use of MSCs can be applied as salvage therapy in refractory chronic GVHD was brought to the agenda with this publication [70]. In another study published in 2014, CR response was obtained in 5 patients and PR response was obtained in 23 patients, while no response was obtained in 10 patients in the 12-month follow-up of 38 chronic GVHD patients after MSC infusion [71]. Recently, in a meta-analysis published by Li et al. in 2021, similar to previous studies, it was shown that co-transplantation of MSCs in HSCT patients facilitated neutrophil and platelet engraftment, reduced the risk of chronic GVHD but did not affect the risk of relapse or mortality [72].

In animal models, it has been demonstrated that MSCs facilitate HSC engraftment and prevent the development of lethal GVHD with their immunomodulatory effects since they are progenitor cells of the bone marrow stroma, and the positive results associated with MSC infusion in humans overlap with these data. However, when the subgroup analyses of these studies were analyzed, it was observed that in children and adolescents who underwent HLA non-identical HSCT due to hematologic malignancy, co-transplantation of MSCs seemed to be the optimal treatment, while in HLA-identical transplant recipients, OS rates were lower in those who received MSC co-infusion compared to those who did not receive. Therefore, HLA-identical transplant recipients should be vigilant in terms of disease relapse after MSC co-infusion [72].

Gao et al. published a phase II, multicenter study investigating the efficacy and safety of post-transplant umbilical cord-derived MSCs in the prophylaxis of chronic GVHD in patients undergoing haploidentical HSCT for hematologic malignancy. The study included 124 patients from five different centers. A mean of two to four MSC infusions were performed, 17 (27.4%) patients in the MSC-infused group developed chronic GVHD, 14 (22.6%) of them had mild/moderate chronic GVHD, 4 (4.8%) patients developed severe chronic GVHD. In the control group who did not receive MSC infusion, 30 patients (48.4%) developed chronic GVHD, 22 (35.5%) of them had mild/moderate chronic GVHD, while 8 (12.9%) patients developed severe chronic GVHD [73]. At the end of the study, 41 patients with and 38 patients without MSC infusion survived, while 37 patients had leukemia relapse and 8 patients had transplant-related mortality due to severe infection. Two-year OS rates were found to be 66.1% in patients who received MSC therapy and 61.3% in those who did not receive MSC infusion and were statistically insignificant [43]. In this study, although there was no change in the number of T cells, an increase in the number of T-reg cells and Th1/Th2 ratio was detected in the patients after the infusion of MSCs. Lei Gao et al. supported that an increase in the number of T-reg cells with MSC infusion decreases the incidence of chronic GVHD with this publication. An increase in Th2 cells is an important factor in increasing fibrosis and an increase in Th2 cells has been shown in chronic GVHD. Again, the decrease in Th2 in the studies of Lei et al. supports the idea that MSC infusion may be effective in preventing the development of chronic GVHD [43, 74].

In another recent 11-patient study by Boberg et al., bone marrow-derived MSC infusions were administered intermittently for a period of 6–12 months and six patients showed a decrease in GVHD-related symptoms and an increase in quality of life. After the infusions, an increase in naive B and T cells and T-reg cell count was detected [75].

In 2015, Peng et al. published a prospective study of 23 patients and as a result of this study, favorable results were obtained with the use of MSCs in patients with refractory chronic GVHD. CR or PR was achieved in 20 of 23 patients with chronic GVHD at 12-month follow-up, and it was that this clinical improvement may be due to an increase in the number of CD5-positive B cells producing IL-10, an immune suppressive cytokine, after MSC infusion [76].

The results of studies on the use of MSC in patients with chronic GVHD have been partially summarized here, and it is clear that more studies are needed to reach a clearer conclusion on the efficacy of MSC in chronic GVHD.

4. Conclusion

There have been many studies on MSC applications in patients with both acute GVHD and chronic GVHD, and as a result of the immunosuppressive and immune modulatory activity of MSCs, there is a majority of opinions supporting the efficacy of MSC infusion in the prevention of GVHD and alleviation of clinical findings. Although the number of studies on acute GVHD is higher than chronic GVHD in the literature, the number of publications on chronic GVHD has been increasing recently and the more the number of studies increases, the more new information is obtained about MSCs. The heterogeneity of the patient populations and the small number of patients in the study groups may be an important factor in the different results of the studies. In addition, the reasons for HSCT, different protocols, heterogeneity in the differentiation capacities of the differentiation capacity of the differentiated MSCs, and the different tissue from which the MSC originates may also explain the differences between the results. There is also a concern about disease relapse related to the use of MSCs due to immune suppression, and the data on this issue are not clear. With the advances in genetic engineering, cellular therapies are now utilized in many diseases and more studies are needed on these therapies. As a result of the widespread use of HSCT in the treatment of malignant/non-malignant hematologic diseases, the increase in the number of centers performing HSCT and the increase in the number of HSCT and the associated increase in the incidence of GVHD, preventing GVHD and reducing GVHD-related mortality and morbidity should be an important health strategy. The studies indicating that the use of MSCs is effective in the prevention and treatment of GVHD are promising, but more and more comprehensive studies on this subject are needed.

Author details

Neslihan Mandacı Şanlı[1*] and Aysu Timuroğlu[2]

1 Erciyes University Hematology Department, Bone Marrow Transplant Center, Kayseri, Turkey

2 Erzurum City Hospital Hematology Department, Erzurum, Turkey

*Address all correspondence to: ortoforia@hotmail.com

IntechOpen

References

[1] Hmadcha A, Martin-Montalvo A, Benoit R, et al. Therapeutic potential of mesenchymal stem cells for cancer therapy. Frontiers in Bioengineering and Biotechnology. 2020;**8**(43):1-13. DOI: 10.3389/fbioe.2020.00043

[2] Mendirattaa M, Mendirattab M, Mohantyb S, et al. Breaking the graft-versus-host-disease barrier: Mesenchymal stromal/stem cells as precision healers. International Reviews of Immunology. 2023;**43**(2):95-112. DOI: 10.1080/08830185.2023.2252007

[3] Merimi M, El-Majzoub R, Lagneaux L, et al. The therapeutic potential of mesenchymal stromal cells for regenerative medicine: Current knowledge and future understandings. Frontiers in Cell and Developmental Biology. 2021;**9**:661532. DOI: 10.3389/fcell.2021.661532

[4] Galipeau J, Sensébé L. Mesenchymal stromal cells: Clinical challenges and therapeutic opportunities. Cell Stem Cell. 2018;**22**(6):824-833. DOI: 10.1016/j.stem.2018.05.004

[5] Hass R, Kasper C, Böhm S, et al. Different populations and sources of human mesenchymal stem cells (MSC): A comparison of adult and neonatal tissue-derived MSC. Cell Communication and Signaling: CCS. 2011;**9**(1):12. DOI: 10.1186/1478-811X-9-12

[6] Ponnaiyan D, Bhat KM, Bhat GS. Comparison of immuno-phenotypes of stem cells from human dental pulp and periodontal ligament. International Journal of Immunopathology and Pharmacology. 2012;**25**(1):127-134. DOI: 10.1177/039463201202500115

[7] Nagamura-Inoue T, He H. Umbilical cord-derived mesenchymal stem cells: Their advantages and potential clinical utility. World Journal of Stem Cells. 2014;**6**(2):195-202. DOI: 10.4252/wjsc.v6.i2.195

[8] Dominici M, Blanc KL, Mueller I, et al. Minimal criteria for defining multipotent mesenchymal stromal cells. The international society for cellular therapy position statement. Cytotherapy. 2006;**8**(4):315-317. DOI: 10.1080/14653240600855905

[9] Escacena N, Quesada-Hernández E, Capilla-Gonzalez V, et al. Bottlenecks in the efficient use of advanced therapy medicinal products based on mesenchymal stromal cells. Stem Cells International. 2015;**895714**:1-12. DOI: 10.1155/2015/895714

[10] Jovic D, Yu Y, Wang D, et al. A brief overview of global trends in MSC-based cell therapy. Stem Cell Reviews and Reports. 2022;**18**:1525-1545. DOI: doi.org/10.1007/s12015-022-10369-1

[11] Beeravolu N, Khan I, McKee C, et al. Isolation and comparative analysis of potential stem/progenitor cells from different regions of human umbilical cord. Stem Cell Research. 2016;**16**:696-711. DOI: 10.1016/j.scr.2016.04.010

[12] Beeravolu N, McKee C, Alamri A, et al. Isolation and characterization of mesenchymal stromal cells from human umbilical cord and fetal placenta. Journal of Visualized Experiments. 2017;**55224**(122):1-13. DOI: 10.3791/55224

[13] Lo B, Parham L. Ethical issues in stem cell research. Endocrine Reviews. 2009;**30**(3):204-213. DOI: 10.1210/er.2008-0031. Epub 2009 Apr 14

[14] Ramos-Zúñiga R, González-Pérez O, Macías-Ornelas A, et al. Ethical implications in the use of embryonic and adult neural stem cells. Stem Cells International. 2012;**470949**:1-7. DOI: 10.1155/2012/470949

[15] Ovalı E. Mezenkimal Kök Hücre Kaynakları ve Üretimi. Türk Hematoloji Derneği Mezenkimal Kök Hücre Kurs Kitabı. Türk Hematoloji Derneği, İzmir; 2008

[16] Lee KD, Kuo TK, Whang-Peng J, et al. In vitro hepatic differentiation of human mesenchymal stem cells. Hepatology. 2004;**40**:1275-1284

[17] Paunescu V, Deak E, Herman D, et al. In vitro differentiation of human mesenchymal stem cells to epithelial lineage. Journal of Cellular and Molecular Medicine. 2007;**11**:502-508

[18] Quevedo HC, Hatzistergos KE, Oskouei BN, et al. Allogeneic mesenchymal stem cells restore cardiac function in chronic ischemic cardiomyopathy via trilineage differentiating capacity. Proceedings. National Academy of Sciences. United States of America. 2009;**106**:14022-14027. DOI: 10.1073

[19] Gervois P, Struys T, Hilkens P, Bronckaers A, et al. Neurogenic maturation of human dental pulp stem cells following neurosphere generation induces morphological and electrophysiological characteristics of functional neurons. Stem Cells and Development. 2015;**24**:296-311. DOI: 10.1089

[20] Salgado AJ, Reis RL, Sousa NJ, et al. Adipose tissue derived stem cells secretome: Soluble factors and their roles in regenerative medicine. Current Stem Cell Research & Therapy. 2010;**5**:103-110. DOI: 10.2174/157488810791268564

[21] Baumrin E, Loren AW, Falk SJ, et al. Chronic graft-versus-host disease. Part I: Epidemiology, pathogenesis, and clinical manifestations. Journal of the American Academy of Dermatology. 2024;**90**(1): 1-16. DOI: 10.1016/j.jaad.2022.12.024

[22] Shafeghat Z, Dorfaki M, Dehrouyeh S, et al. Mesenchymal stem cell-derived exosomes for managing graft-versus-host disease: An updated view. Transplant Immunology. 2023;**81**:101957. DOI: 10.1016/j.trim.2023.101957

[23] Zhao L, Chen S, Yang P, et al. The role of mesenchymal stem cells in hematopoietic stem cell transplantation: Prevention and treatment of graft-versushost disease. Stem Cell Research & Therapy. 2019;**10**:182

[24] Aladağ E, Kelkitli E, Göker H. Acute graft-versus-host disease: A brief review. Turkish Journal of Hematology. 2020;**37**:1-4

[25] Flowers ME, Inamoto Y, Carpenter PA, et al. Comparative analysis of risk factors for acute graft-versus-host disease and for chronic graft-versus-host disease according to national institutes of health consensus criteria. Blood. 2011;**117**(11):3214-3219

[26] Jagasia MH, Greinix HT, Arora M, et al. National institutes of health consensus development project on criteria for clinical trials in chronic graft-versus-host disease: I. The 2014 diagnosis and staging working group report. Biology of Blood and Marrow Transplantation. 2015;**21**(3):389-401

[27] Goker H, Haznedaroglu IC, Chao NJ. Acute graft-vs-host disease: Pathobiology and management. Experimental Hematology. 2001;**29**:259-277

[28] Filipovich AH, Weisdorf D, Pavletic S, et al. National Institutes of

Health consensus development project on criteria for clinical trials in chronic graft-versus-host disease: I. Diagnosis and staging working group report. Biology of Blood and Marrow Transplantation. 2005;**11**:945-956

[29] Arora M, Pidala J, Cutler CS, et al. Impact of prior acute GVHD on chronic GVHD outcomes: A chronic graft versus host disease consortium study. Leukemia. 2013;**27**(5):1196-1201

[30] Murata M, Teshima T. Treatment of steroid-refractory acute graft-versus-host disease using commercial mesenchymal stem cell products. Frontiers in Immunology. 2021;**12**:724380

[31] Ankrum JA, Ong JF, Karp JM. Mesenchymal stem cells: Immune evasive, not immune privileged. Nature Biotechnology. 2014;**32**:252-260

[32] Huang Y, Wu Q, Tam PKH. Immunomodulatory mechanisms of mesenchymal stem cells and their potential clinical applications. International Journal of Molecular Sciences. 2022;**23**:10023

[33] Spaggiari GM, Capobianco A, Becchetti S, et al. Mesenchymal stem cell-natural killer cell interactions: Evidence that activated NK cells are capable of killing MSCs, whereas MSCs can inhibit IL-2-induced NK-cell proliferation. Blood. 2006;**107**:1484-1490

[34] Di Nicola M, Carlo-Stella C, Magni M, et al. Human bone marrow stromal cells suppress T-lymphocyte proliferation induced by cellular or nonspecific mitogenic stimuli. Blood. 2002;**99**:3838-3843

[35] Majumdar MK, Keane-Moore M, Buyaner D, et al. Characterization and functionality of cell surface molecules on human mesenchymal stem cells. Journal of Biomedical Science. 2003;**10**:228-241

[36] Ren G, Zhao X, Zhang L, et al. Inflammatory cytokine-induced intercellular adhesion molecule-1 and vascular cell adhesion molecule-1 in mesenchymal stem cells are critical for immunosuppression. Journal of Immunology. 2010;**184**:2321-2328

[37] Sakaguchi S, Yamaguchi T, Nomura T, et al. Regulatory T cells and immune tolerance. Cell. 2008;**133**:775-787

[38] Gieseke F, Kruchen A, Tzaribachev N, et al. Proinflammatory stimuli induce galectin-9 in human mesenchymal stromal cells to suppress T-cell proliferation. European Journal of Immunology. 2013;**43**:2741-2749

[39] Cao X, Duan L, Hou H, et al. IGF-1C hydrogel improves the therapeutic effects of MSCs on colitis in mice through PGE2-mediated M2 macrophage polarization. Theranostics. 2020;**10**:7697-7709

[40] Kanakry CG, Fuchs EJ, Luznik L. Modern approaches to HLA-haploidentical blood or marrow transplantation. Nature Reviews. Clinical Oncology. 2016;**13**(2):132

[41] Welniak LA, Blazar BR, Murphy WJ. Immunobiology of allogeneic hematopoietic stem cell transplantation. Annual Review of Immunology. 2007;**25**:139-170

[42] Martin PJ, Rizzo JD, Wingard JR, et al. First- and second-line systemic treatment of acute graft-versus-host disease: Recommendations of the American Society of Blood and Marrow Transplantation. Biology of Blood and Marrow Transplantation. 2012;**18**(8):1150-1163

[43] Gao L, Zhang Y, Hu B, et al. Phase II multicenter, randomized, double-blind

controlled study of efficacy and safety of umbilical cord-derived mesenchymal stromal cells in the prophylaxis of chronic graft-versus-host disease after HLA-haploidentical stem-cell transplantation. Journal of Clinical Oncology. 2016;**34**(24):2843-2850

[44] Cahn JY, Klein JP, Lee SJ, et al. Prospective evaluation of 2 acute graft-versus-host (GVHD) grading systems: A joint Societe Francaise de Greffe de Moelle et Therapie Cellulaire (SFGM-TC), Dana Farber cancer institute (DFCI), and international bone marrow transplant registry (IBMTR) prospective study. Blood. 2005;**106**(4):1495-1500

[45] Uccelli A, Moretta L, Pistoia V. Immunoregulatory function of mesenchymal stem cells. European Journal of Immunology. 2006;**36**(10):2566-2573

[46] Fierabracci A, Del FA, Muraca M, et al. The use of mesenchymal stem cells for the treatment of autoimmunity: From animals models to human disease. Current Drug Targets. 2016;**17**(2):229-238

[47] Kelly K, Rasko JEJ. Mesenchymal stromal cells for the treatment of graft versus host disease. Frontiers in Immunology. 2021;**12**:761616

[48] Liu S, Liu F, Zhou Y, et al. Immunosuppressive property of MSCs mediated by cell surface receptors. Frontiers in Immunology. 2020;**11**:1076

[49] Matula Z, Németh A, Lőrincz P, et al. The role of extracellular vesicle and tunneling nanotube-mediated intercellular cross-talk between mesenchymal stem cells and human peripheral T cells. Stem Cells and Development. 2016;**25**(23):1818-1832

[50] Li H, Wang C, He T, et al. Mitochondrial transfer from bone marrow mesenchymal stem cells to motor neurons in spinal cord injury rats via gap junction. Theranostics. 2019;**9**(7):2017-2035

[51] Bernardo ME, Fibbe WE. Mesenchymal stromal cells: Sensors and switchers of inflammation. Cell Stem Cell. 2013;**13**(4):392-402

[52] Galleu A, Riffo-Vasquez Y, Trento C, et al. Apoptosis in mesenchymal stromal cells induces in vivo recipient-mediated immunomodulation. Science Translational Medicine. 2017;**9**(416):1-11

[53] Cheung TS, Bertolino GM, Giacomini C, et al. Mesenchymal stromal cells for graft versus host disease: Mechanism-based biomarkers. Frontiers in Immunology. 2020;**11**:1338

[54] Cheung TS, Galleu A, von Bonin M, Bornhäuser M, Dazzi F. Apoptotic mesenchymal stromal cells induce prostaglandin E2 in monocytes: Implications for the monitoring of mesenchymal stromal cell activity. Haematologica. 2019;**104**(10):e438-e441

[55] Bartholomew A, Sturgeon C, Siatskas M, et al. Mesenchymal stem cells suppress lymphocyte proliferation in vitro and prolong skin graft survival in vivo. Experimental Hematology. 2002;**30**(1):42-48

[56] Dazzi F, Ramasamy R, Glennie S, et al. The role of mesenchymal stem cells in haemopoiesis. Blood Reviews. 2006;**20**(3):161-171

[57] Devine SM, Hoffman R. Role of mesenchymal stem cells in hematopoietic stem cell transplantation. Current Opinion in Hematology. 2000;**7**(6):358-363

[58] Kuzmina LA, Petinati NA, Parovichnikova EN, et al. Multipotent

mesenchymal stromal cells for the prophylaxis of acute graft-versus-host disease-a phase II study. Stem Cells International. 2012;**1**:968213

[59] Blanc KL et al. Treatment of severe acute graft-versushost disease with third party haploidentical mesenchymal stem cells. Lancet. 2004;**363**:1439-1441

[60] Kebriaei P, Isola L, Bahceci E, et al. Adult human mesenchymal stem cells added to corticosteroid therapy for the treatment of acute graft-versus-host disease. Biology of Blood and Marrow Transplantation. 2009;**15**(7):804-811

[61] Soder RP, Dawn B, Weiss ML, et al. A phase I study to evaluate two doses of Wharton's jelly-derived mesenchymal stromal cells for the treatment of De novo high-risk or steroid-refractory acute graft versus host disease. Stem Cell Reviews and Reports. 2020;**16**(5):979-991

[62] Muroi K, Miyamura K, Okada M, et al. Bone marrow-derived mesenchymal stem cells (JR-031) for steroid-refractory grade III or IV acute graft-versus-host disease: A phase II/III study. International Journal of Hematology. 2015;**103**:243-250

[63] Baron F, Lechanteur C, Willems E, et al. Cotransplantation of mesenchymal stem cells might prevent death from graft-versus-host disease (GVHD) without abrogating graft-versus-tumor effects after HLA-mismatched allogeneic transplantation following nonmyeloablative conditioning. Biology of Blood and Marrow Transplantation. 2010;**16**:838-847

[64] Galipeau J. The mesenchymal stromal cells dilemma--does a negative phase III trial of random donor mesenchymal stromal cells in steroid-resistant graft-versushost disease represent a death knell or a bump in the road? Cytotherapy. 2013;**15**:2-8

[65] Ning H, Yang F, Jiang M, et al. The correlation between cotransplantation of mesenchymal stem cells and higher recurrence rate in hematologic malignancy patients: Outcome of a pilot clinical study. Leukemia. 2008;**22**(3):593-599

[66] Liu K, Chen Y, Zeng Y, et al. Coinfusion of mesenchymal stromal cells facilitates platelet recovery without increasing leukemia recurrence in haploidentical hematopoietic stem cell transplantation: A randomized, controlled clinical study. Stem Cells and Development. 2011;**20**(10):1679-1685

[67] Doglio M, Crossland RE, Alho AC, et al. Cell-based therapy in prophylaxis and treatment of chronic graft-versus-host disease. Frontiers in Immunology. 2022;**13**:1045168

[68] Liu X, Wu M, Peng Y, et al. Improvement in poor graft function after allogeneic hematopoietic stem cell transplantation upon administration of mesenchymal stem cells from third-party donors: A pilot prospective study. Cell Transplantation. 2014;**23**(9):1087-1098

[69] Morata-Tarifa C., Macías-Sánchez M.D.M., Gutiérrez-Pizarraya A., et al. Mesenchymal stromal cells for the prophylaxis and treatment of graft-versus-host disease-a meta-analysis. Stem Cell Research & Therapy. 2020;**11**(1):64,1-12 DOI: 10.1186/s13287-020-01592-z

[70] Weng JY, Du X, Geng SX, et al. Mesenchymal stem cell as salvage treatment for refractory chronic GVHD. Bone Marrow Transplantation. 2010;**45**:1732-1740

[71] Peng Y, Chen X, Liu Q, et al. Alteration of Na¨ıve and memory B-cell subset in chronic graft-versus-host disease patients after treatment

with mesenchymal stromal cells.
Stem Cells Translational Medicine.
2014;**3**(9):1023-1031

[72] Li T, Luo C, Zhang J, et al. Efficacy
and safety of mesenchymal stem cells
co-infusion in allogeneic hematopoietic
stem cell transplantation: A systematic
review and meta-analysis. Stem Cell
Research & Therapy. 2021;**12**(1):246

[73] Zhang C, Gao L, Zhu L, et al. Phase
II multicenter, randomized, double-blind
controlled study of efficacy and safety
of umbilical cord–derived mesenchymal
stromal cells in the prophylaxis of
chronic graft-versus-host disease
after HLA-haploidentical stem-cell
transplantation. Journal of Clinical
Oncology. 2016;**34**(24):2843-2845

[74] Kim J, Choi WS, Kim HJ, et al.
Prevention of chronic graft-versus-
host disease by stimulation with
glucocorticoid-induced TNF receptor.
Experimental & Molecular Medicine.
2006;**38**:94-99

[75] Boberg E, Bahr L, Afram G, et al.
Treatment of chronic GvHD with
mesenchymal stromal cells induces
durable responses: A phase II study.
Stem Cells Translational Medicine.
2020;**9**:1190-1202

[76] Peng Y, Chen X, Liu Q, et al.
Mesenchymal stromal cells infusions
improve refractory chronic graft versus
host disease through an increase of CD5+
regulatory B cells producing interleukin
10. Leukemia. 2015;**29**(3):636-646

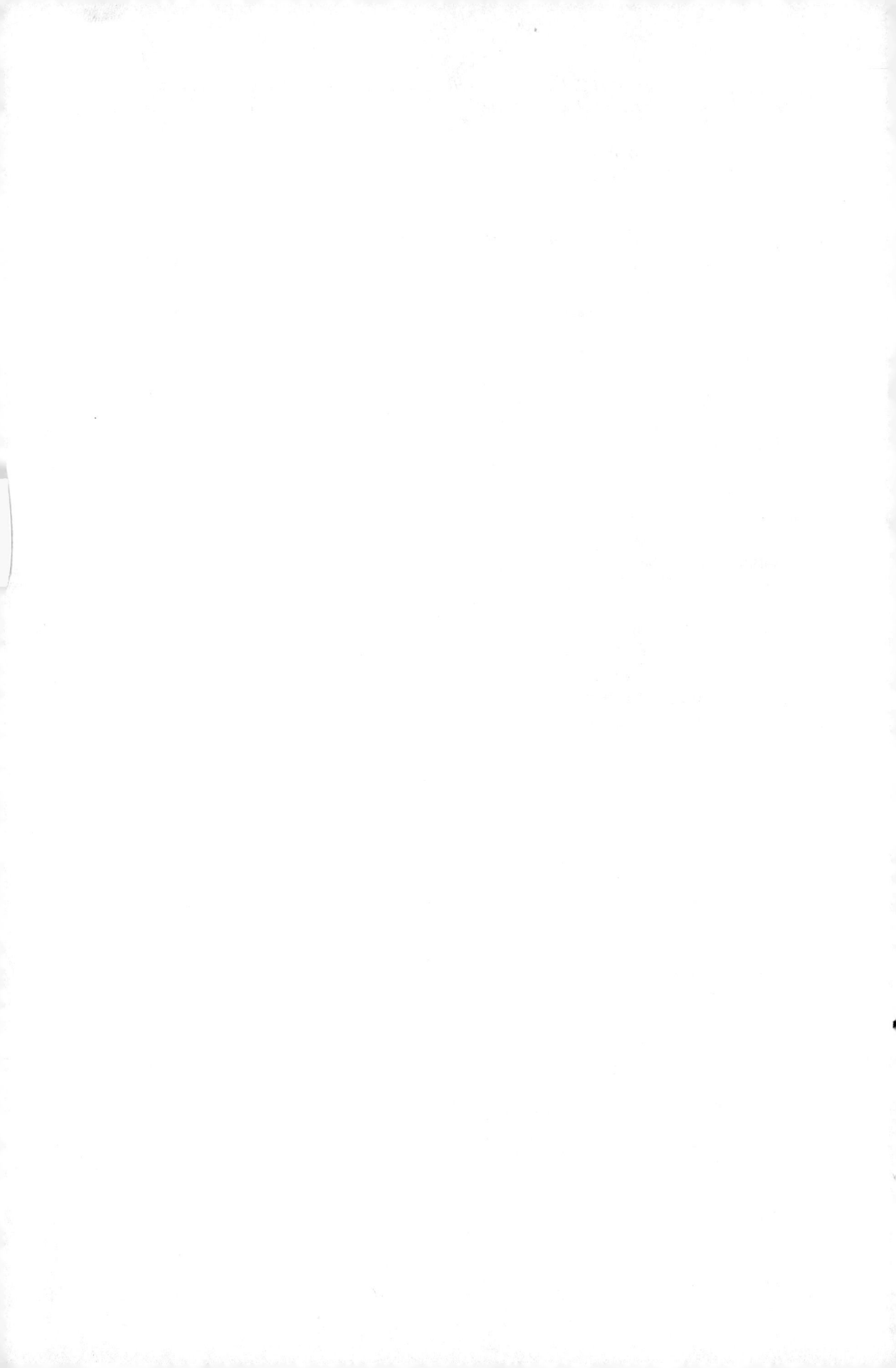